A LOVE OF LIFE
The story of Sarah Hotter

A LOVE OF LIFE
THE STORY OF SARAH HOTTER

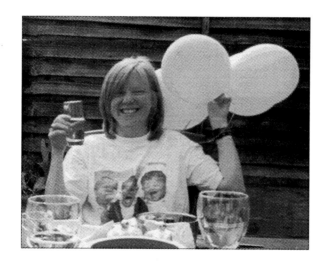

KEN VEITCH

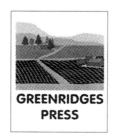

**GREENRIDGES
PRESS**

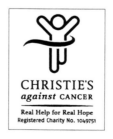

CHRISTIE'S
against CANCER

Real Help for Real Hope
Registered Charity No. 1049751

All profits from the sale of this book go to the Christie Hospital, Manchester

ISBN 1 902019 05 9
First published December 2002

Published by:
Greenridges Press
an imprint of
Anne Loader Publications
13 Vale Road, Hartford,
Northwich, Cheshire CW8 1PL
Gt Britain
Tel: 01606 75660   Fax: 01606 77609
e-mail: anne@leoniepress.com
Website: www.anneloaderpublications.co.uk
www.leoniepress.com

Printed by:
Anne Loader Publications

Cover photograph:
Sarah celebrates her 32nd birthday, May 1998

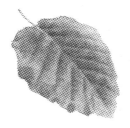

For the family and friends of
SARAH LOUISE HOTTER
10 May 1966 - 25 December 1999

Que Dios la tenga en su gloria

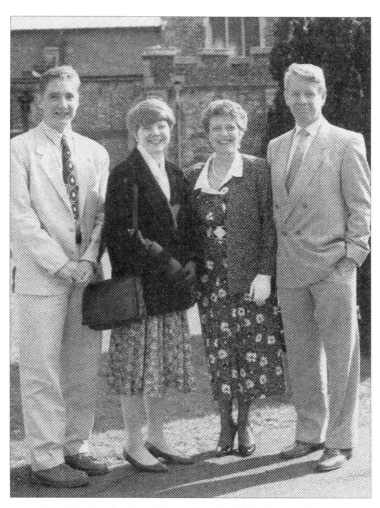

The Hotter family: Mark, Sarah, Valerie and Bruce

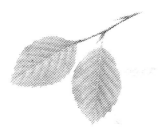

AUTHOR'S NOTE

I WISH to thank everyone who helped in any way with the compilation of this book. When Valerie and Mark agreed that the story of Sarah should be written, we contacted the very wide circle of her family and friends. The circle included people who first knew Sarah professionally, and who became her friends because of the special rapport she was able to create with them.

Everyone we contacted responded with enthusiasm, and their contributions, written with much care, show how the love that Sarah gave out was, and still is, reflected back to her. I am sorry it has not been possible to include every contribution.

I particularly wish to thank Sarah's mother Valerie and her brother Mark for their kind and constant support and for allowing me to use their family papers.

Thanks also to Anne and Jack Loader, Greenridges Press, Hartford, Northwich and to the Christie Hospital, Manchester, for their encouragement.

I am a child of the typewriter and the Roneo ink duplicator; without the patience and the computer expertise of my daughter Mary this book would have remained 'just an idea'. To her also, I am most grateful.

KV

One has just to be oneself.
That's my basic message.
The moment you accept yourself as you are,
All burdens, all mountains, simply disappear.
Then life is a sheer joy, a festival of lights

Bagwan Shree Rajneesh

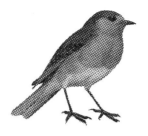

CONTENTS

FOREWORD
Sister Tina Johnson

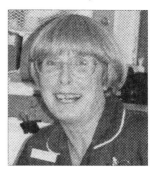

THIS book is a tribute to Sarah Hotter. Sarah's life was one brimming with vitality and enthusiasm in all she did.

You will find how she touched lives with her own love of life and her concern for other people. The willingness of such a diverse group of people to express their feelings and share treasured memories is testament to the love, affection and respect that they still hold for Sarah. Many remain enriched by their contact with her.

It was my privilege to participate in Sarah's care in hospital leading up to her death. It is my loss not to have known her before. I would like to pay tribute also to Sarah's mother Val, and her brother Mark. Their untiring care and devotion to Sarah over the last few days was an example to us all. They made it possible for a loved daughter and sister to 'play it her way' right up to the end. I know this was appreciated by Sarah.

This book will, I hope, challenge you to live life to the full. Read, enjoy, and go for Quality of Life too!

• *Tina Johnson has been Sister of Ward 3 at the Christie Hospital for the last four years. After qualifying as a nurse from the South Manchester Health Authority and a brief spell on the Renal Unit at Withington Hospital in Manchester, she has worked at the Christie Hospital for almost fourteen years.*

AUTHOR'S PREFACE

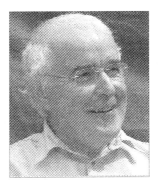

IN 1996 I was the Head of Beeston Outdoor Education Centre, a former village school halfway between Nantwich and Chester, beautifully situated among farms and woodland, and only half a mile from the famous medieval castle of Beeston. The school had closed in 1969, and been converted by the Cheshire Education Authority for use as a short-stay residential centre. Its visitors were mainly children in the 5-11 age range, whose teachers would bring their classes for two nights at a time; ideal for exploring the surrounding countryside, and learning to live together!

One afternoon I received a telephone call from the newly-appointed Education Officer at the Northwich Salt Museum. Could she visit me to find out more about the outdoor education and museums service? An appointment was made.

So it was that I first met Sarah Hotter on the car park at Beeston. We 'clicked' immediately and by the time we sat down in my office about a minute later, I felt I was conversing with a friend I had known for years. Without making any effort to impress, Sarah shone out as a singularly colourful person, and not just on account of that beautiful hair! She was attractive, witty, wise, and bright in the fullest sense of that word and she carried these qualities in a natural easy sort of way. I had told my staff that we were to have a 'working meeting'. They told me all they heard was laughter! Sarah returned to her duties, and did them very well. But she had hardly got into her stride when she was stricken in the spring of 1998 with the brain tumour that was to prove fatal.

I visited Sarah and her mother Val on several occasions during Sarah's eighteen-month illness. The love they showed for each other, the calm practical way they dealt with Sarah's steady deterioration, and their never-failing humour and consideration for others – notwithstanding all the painful times they must have experienced – are things indelibly stamped on my mind, and on the minds of everybody who knew Sarah.

Sarah was a 'people' person, comfortable with those of any age or walk of life. At Northwich she helped to produce a book telling the story of Nellie Osborne, a lady whose life gives a very interesting insight into local social history. It occurred to me that the story of Sarah should be told too. I put the idea to Val and after due thought she and Sarah's brother Mark decided we should go ahead. Val put me in touch with people whose lives were touched by Sarah's. Every one of them has been happy to contribute their recollections of Sarah.

The Christie Hospital in Manchester, where Sarah spent her final days, has given its official authorisation to this book. All profits from our sales will be donated to the Christie.

The first part of the story describes Sarah's life, from 1966 to her death in 1999. The second part contains recollections of Sarah by her family and friends. When Val invited these recollections she said: "Try to jot something down as it occurs to you, not 'essays'; just quick jottings, thoughts, somewhere you may have gone together, a party maybe, a dinner out somewhere, what you may have done together; any little things."

Val's request elicited a lot of offerings, which show the depth and breadth of Sarah's personality. These have been arranged mainly in the final section of the book; others are in the earlier parts of the story.

What made Sarah tick? Many have spoken of the fun they had with Sarah, her dependability, her adventurousness, her high intelligence, her determination, her deep personal faith and her vocation of care for others, shown all through her thirty three years and never more so than when she knew her earthly life would soon be ending.

Sarah was a modest person. She never trumpeted her achievements. She had a strong social conscience. She was a Socialist in the truest sense of the word and she lived what she believed. She was an active member of Amnesty International. She would talk about political prisoners and she did her best to support Amnesty in its work, by doing house-to-house collections and writing letters to governments, seeking the release of prisoners of conscience.

Sarah's sense of fun and of the ridiculous was strong. There would be gales of laughter in the Hotter household – the loud raucous outrageous Brown laugh – as many a silly moment was shared, with Bruce looking on in gentle amusement at the dottiness of his wife, daughter and son.

Sarah belonged to a remarkable, lively and loving family, and her character was such that she was able to draw out courage, calmness and humour abundantly in the people whose lives she touched. This is a story of hope, and as Val emphasises, "Sarah was fun and laughter above all else".

The last two pages give us a Celtic benediction (a favourite prayer of Sarah and Val) then Sarah signs off with a characteristic command.

I am not sure that this story has an 'end' at all. The hope of all of us who wrote it is, in the words of her surgeon, that others in similar circumstances will be able to draw strength from Sarah's life and all that came from it. I chose the title 'A Love of Life' because Sarah was an enthusiast in everything she did. The word enthusiasm derives from the Greek word *'entheos'*, 'possessed by a god, inspired'.

I think this describes Sarah absolutely.

Ken Veitch
Nantwich
August 2002

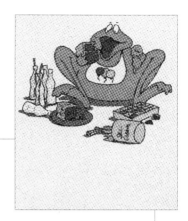

Dear Mummy,

HAPPY BURSTDAY!

Freak out! Let your hair down!

Eat a potato!

After all — you're not THAT fat!

Lots of love,

Sarah
xx

From Sarah to Val around 1983.
© 1981 Thought Factory; published by The Paper House Ltd., Northleach

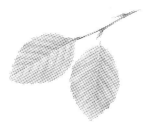

Chapter 1
ATLANTIC VOYAGES
1961 – 1964

Roam abroad in the world, and take thy fill of its enjoyments
before the day shall come when thou must quit it for good

Sa'di, Gulistan, 1258

IN March 1961 the Royal Mail ship *Aragon* left Buenos Aires, Argentina, bound for Tilbury, London, with a cargo of chilled meat and several hundred passengers.

Among the passengers, and travelling with two friends in Third Class, "two feet above the propellers", was Valerie Brown. With his wife and family Valerie's great grandfather Michael Furlong, formerly of Wexford, had emigrated to Argentina to work for a company that bred horses in a farming area close to Buenos Aires familiarly known as 'El Campo', or 'The Camp'. Great-grandfather Brown from Kent, Grandfather Joyce from London, great-grandmother Laclau from the Basque region of France, and the Furlongs, were soon integrated into the sizeable British community.

It was the done thing for people like Valerie, holder of a British passport, to spend time in Britain and other parts of Europe on a working holiday. Valerie's plan was to be away for one year. She had never been out of Argentina before, and she was thoroughly looking forward to her great adventure. Happy with her friends,

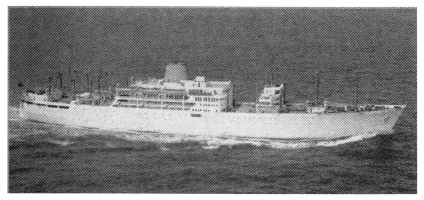

Royal Mail Lines 'Aragon', 20,000 tons

she felt no trepidation at all. She had been saving for two years to pay for this trip.

The voyage up the Atlantic would take three weeks. But before they had travelled far, the group was invited into the cabins of the ship's officers. Among these was Bruce Hotter, one of the Navigating Officers of the *Aragon*. He had already espied the three girls from his vantage position as they boarded the ship. They met a few times with Bruce and his colleagues during the voyage to England.

Arriving at Tilbury a month later, the group went by taxi to their pre-booked hostel near Hyde Park Gate. Val remembers how big London seemed, and how strange it was to hear everyone speaking English and to see signs in English. When Val and her friend Florence told their taxi driver they had come from Argentina to visit England he said, "Well, Miss, you'll find it's very much home from home."

The next morning a note arrived at the hostel. It was addressed to "Val". Hereafter, Val recalls, Bruce always addressed her as "Valerie". The note requested Val to telephone Bruce (Val still remembers the number). Bruce's father was the manager of Lloyd's Bank in Hertford, near London. Val and her two friends went to tea with Bruce's parents, followed by an outing to Luton Hoo, then a meal. Much later, Val found out that Bruce's father had told him: "I know which one you've got your eye on!"

Bruce's sister Ann remembers their early days:

"Bruce and I were both born in Gillingham, Kent and lived there until August 1939 when we went to Walmer, Kent, to stay with Mummy's parents and Auntie Gladys. I think we used to stay all month and Daddy would come down for his two weeks holiday. Gillingham is part of the 'Medway Towns'; the other towns being Chatham, which had a big naval dockyard and Rochester, which had a flying boat factory. Daddy worked in Chatham. The towns were right on the flight path from France to London and were surrounded by fighter stations, so I assume everyone felt we would be safer in Walmer. However, Walmer was two miles from the coast at Deal. The winter of 1939-1940 was very, very cold and snowy. The sea froze at Deal. A ship went right through the middle of the pier one night and there were German landmines on the beach. Bruce used to cry when the sirens went. I can remember us blowing toy trumpets to distract him but it didn't work. I went to a convent school for six months which was awful; the only time in my life that I hated school. In the winter Grandpa died of a stroke. I wasn't told until after the funeral. Grown-ups didn't discuss things with children in those days.

"Meanwhile plans had been made for Mummy and us two, plus Auntie Phyl and her two children, to live in a rented house in Wotton-Under-Edge, Gloucestershire. Apparently we were in Dover station when troops rescued from Dunkirk were coming through. We eventually arrived at the house late at night and it didn't have electricity! Gas lighting only. Actually for children it was a lovely area in which to live; on the edge of a small town with the countryside, including lovely beechwoods all around. We were 20 miles from Bristol and one night it was so badly bombed the whole house was shaking. Fathers used to come for the weekend about once a month. Daddy used to bring all the sweeties he could get hold of, by walking home and going into every little shop. During this period he boarded with the parents of one of his fellow bank clerks who had gone into the navy.

"In 1942 it was considered safer for us to return to Kent and we went to live in Rochester at which time I went to Rochester Grammar School and Bruce went to a local Elementary school. Then the doodlebugs started and later the V2s which were scarier because you never heard them. Bruce and I and the cat used to sleep in the air raid shelter until Bruce and I got bad colds. Bruce went to King's School, Rochester for our last two years there. We moved to Hertford in 1948 in the first family car after Daddy had been made Manager of Lloyds Bank in that town."

From then on, Bruce and Val met every two months, fitting in with Bruce's duties at sea. In between times, Val enjoyed life in London with her friends. By Christmas 1961 she was beginning to feel "there's definitely something in this". Christmas was spent with friends of Val's mother at a smart hotel in Bournemouth. The possibility of Val staying in England was discussed. Her return passage to Buenos Aires was booked for March 1962. She cancelled it. This was Val's first "big decision". She can't recall her parents' reaction, but now as a parent herself she can imagine how difficult it must have been for them, the more so as she didn't talk with them all that much, relying instead on letters. Overseas telephone calls were expensive.

Having spent her spare cash soon after arriving in England, Val took a job with Vickers Ltd., the engineering and shipbuilding firm. She used her skills in Spanish and shorthand-typing, and found a flat to live in. She shared this flat with five local girls.

One evening in September 1962 Bruce asked Val to marry him. They became engaged but decided not to marry until Bruce had gained his Master's Ticket, entitling him to the command of a ship. Bruce's and Val's time together was limited for the present. Bruce remained at sea for lengthy periods, continuing to work as a Navigating Officer on Royal Mail ships, mainly on the South American route. He duly qualified to be a Captain, but was being held back by the 'dead men's shoes' principle. Captains' posts were few and far between, and the Royal Mail Company was contracting because of the availability of cheaper and easier air travel.

Val did have to return to Argentina in 1963. A telegram had arrived from her father with the news that Val's mother was very ill. Val had to leave immediately. She called the Royal Mail office to contact Bruce, who was just about to sail from Liverpool. Bruce arranged for his parents to come to Val, and Bruce's father provided the cash (later repaid by Val's father) for her journey back

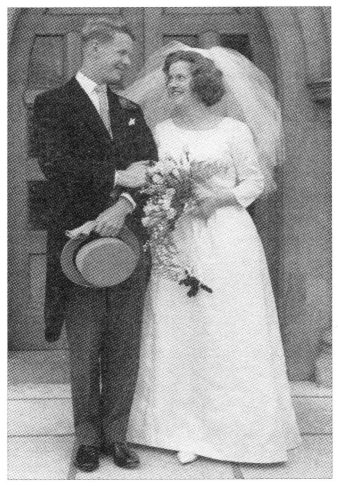

The marriage of Bruce Hotter and Valerie Brown, 9 May 1964
(Photo: W J L Longland, Shepperton, Middlesex)

to Buenos Aires. She arrived there on 21 May 1963, ten days before her mother died. She remained for a few weeks in Argentina before returning to England.

The wedding of Bruce Hotter and Valerie Brown took place on 9 May 1964 at St Ignatius Roman Catholic Church, Sunbury on Thames, Middlesex. By now Val had established her right of residency in Britain. Val's father and sister travelled from Argentina to attend. Val wished at the time that she could have married in Argentina where all her family lived, and where weddings are, in her words, so jolly and relaxed, with three ceremonies often taking place during the evening in the same church, with the choir singing the same repertoire of hymns. All the guests mingle happily, asking "which wedding are you here for?"

Val had cousins in Sunbury. They acted as her sponsors and she married from their house.

Bruce still continued his work at sea, being away for about two months at a time. But this would not be for long. He and Val bought a house in Eythorne Close, Ashford, Kent, twelve miles from Bruce's parents who had by now moved to Kent. Val was glad to spend some time with them while Bruce was away. Bruce had met Val's parents in 1962, two months after the engagement. Val had let them know that she was betrothed to "a very nice bloke". Val's father told her that as the ship slipped into the dock and Bruce's face appeared above the railings, her mother's face relaxed too; any anxieties were dispelled! A lavish buffet was prepared, to welcome and entertain the family on board. Bruce was a very popular host for Valerie's female cousins when they visited him on the ship.

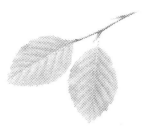

Chapter 2
ASHFORD, KENT
1964 – 1975

Children are entitled to their otherness, and when we reach them it is generally on a point of sheer delight, to us so astonishing, but to them so natural

Alastair Reid, 1963

BRUCE resigned his job in late 1965. He was unhappy to be parted from Val, and knew that the future of the Royal Mail Shipping Company, and that of the Merchant Navy in general, was uncertain. Air services were supplanting ships increasingly. By this time Val was pregnant with their first child. She was not as well as she could wish, and dependent on neighbours for any immediate help, a situation which Bruce and Val both found distressing.

Bruce's new job was as a cheque sorter operator with Barclay's Bank in London. He was to work in London for nine years, commuting from Ashford by main line trains, the Tube, and on foot. This travelling took up three and a half hours per day.

On 10 May 1966 Val's and Bruce's first child, a girl, was born in the maternity wing of Kench Hill Nursing Home at Tenterden in Kent. They named her Sarah Louise. Val thought her baby was beautiful at first sight. In those days, fathers were not encouraged to be present at the birth of a baby. Bruce was sitting waiting at his parents' house, appearing to read a book but without turning any

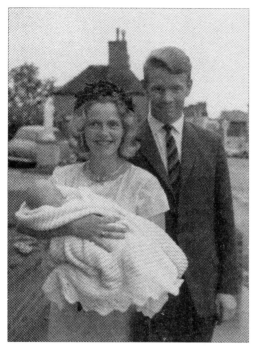

Sarah's christening in July 1966. Val's sister remarked, on seeing the photos: "How English – all the hats!"

pages! A friend who came to see mother and baby thought Val looked like a Cheshire cat. Val said she felt like a Beethoven or a Mozart. Both parents were elated.

Sarah and her brother Mark were both born at Kench Hill Nursing Home. It had an NHS maternity wing, so there were "both ends of the spectrum", the very young and the old, mingling happily together. When Sarah was born and Bruce saw her for the first time, he spent some time counting her toes. He made it six on each foot, both times... the excitement of his first child was obviously too much for him!

Sarah was brought home after nine days. She was a happy baby, a great smiler. She ate lustily, Val recalls, "putting on weight like a trooper". She had a Silver Cross pram with big wheels.

When Mark was born Bruce took Sarah to the hospital. Sarah peered most interestedly down into the carry-cot and bent down to give her little brother a kiss. When he was a little older she would translate Mark's baby gurgles and first attempts at speaking, most efficiently, always getting to his needs before Val could: "Mark wants this, Mummy, or that, Mummy." Sarah and Mark spent endless happy hours playing together. Mark would go into her room and beg for a story. She would pretend to be asleep, but when her eyelids were prised open she would relent and Bruce and Val would go into the room to see her jabbering away at some story or other, with Mark sitting beside her, eyes wide, mouth sometimes ajar, listening intently. Sarah was not above biffing Mark now and then if he seemed insubordinate!

When she was three, Sarah joined the local playgroup for morning sessions two or three times a week. She mixed well with other children and soon had lots of little friends. One day she decided to visit one of these friends without telling Val, and wandered off down the road. She was missing for two hours. A tearful and shaking Val eventually found her having fun in the friend's house, Sarah having said her Mummy knew where she was.

On her own, Sarah enjoyed her books and dollies. She had Lego, but was not all that dexterous.

In September 1971 Sarah started school at St Teresa's RC Primary in Ashford. The Hotters had meanwhile moved to their second home in Ashford, in Canterbury Road, facing the cemetery. Val recalls how police came with torches one dark night because the local witches' coven was dancing on the gravestones.

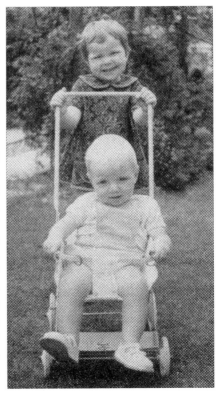

Sarah made a flying start at school. The teacher in her second class was soon running out of things to teach her and her academic bent was very soon apparent. Sarah became an avid reader, and Val and Bruce read constantly to her also. Among her favourite stories were Puff the Magic Dragon, and Trolls on the Bridge, plus Rupert Bear, fairy stories and nursery rhymes. Sarah also enjoyed drawing, colouring and writing. Val walked Sarah to school, along

Sarah and Mark

9

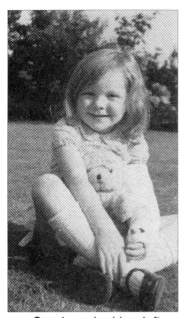

Sarah sucked her left thumb until she broke her arm when she fell off the dining room table in July 1971 – the other one 'wouldn't do', so that was the end of thumb-sucking!

with Mark in his push-chair.

St Teresa's Church was next door to the school. There were many church and school fairs. Everyone worked hard to make these a success. The local church didn't have much money, nor did the school, so it was all hands to the pump and the atmosphere of people mingling and working happily together was something to really remember. The Hotters used to run the toy stall at the school fairs and in general. By the time the family moved to Altrincham in 1975, fairs had become very much of a family thing. On one occasion Val was not sure whether she could make it to one particular fair. There was a LOUD howl of dismay from Sarah: "Oh, Mummy, do come. You're EVER such fun at fairs!" Val dropped everything and went.

St Teresa's in Ashford was a good lively parish, with lots of social events. Parents got on well together and there was easy informal access to the teachers. The parents would collect the children after school – the little ones would tumble out in their blue jackets and skirts or trousers, all looking much the same. On one occasion a parent remarked to Val, "Look at them, they all look the same – one could just pick the nearest hand and take it home to have tea!" Val and her friend Frances Turner would walk their children home.

Sarah related well to both children and adults. Val and Bruce liked to invite friends to their home, and Sarah fitted in well with them. But there were times when she became upset at not having her own way. One day when Sarah arrived home screaming in rage, Val stuck her under the shower to cool her down. It made no difference; Sarah continued to scream!

Sarah's childhood is remembered by family friends Frances Turner, Sheila Whitelegg, Tessa Flood and Beth ('Auntie Beff') Crump:

Frances Turner writes:

"I remember eight-year-old Sarah reading in St Teresa's Church one Christmas, and being so composed and confident above her years. She read beautifully. As we had a very long garden we used to have bonfire parties at which the Hotters would join us, along with other neighbours, the Sparkes and the Wallages. I can remember it being such fun. The girls always held sparklers.

"Sarah and my daughter Louise attended the Margaret Giles School of Ballet Dancing held in the Parish Rooms. Margaret Giles played the piano. She was a funny old-fashioned spinster with a 'rat-like' dog who went everywhere with her! The ballet teacher was Mrs Taylor who was very strict. This was not a suitable dancing school for either Sarah or Louise who liked to thump about; it was really very sedate and not at all fun.

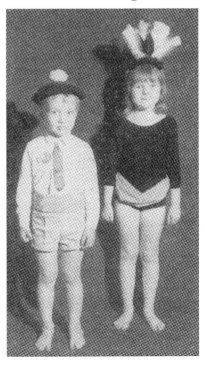

"So we enrolled them both in 'Auntie Betty's Dancing School' which was primarily tap-dancing. They both loved it. They still wore their ballet togs but had bright red tap shoes. And by jove did they tap! They had such fun there. It was a bit disorganised at times and unbelievably noisy, but they could thump and tap to their hearts' content.

"I don't know whether you remember, Valerie, that Auntie Betty also ran a dance class for mothers (you and I did not join in

Mark and Sarah in "Cabaret" performed by Auntie Betty's Dancing Class, around 1974

11

– we preferred to be spectators) I remember one concert that the girls were in and the mothers performed afterwards. Auntie Betty, who was a big lady (and that's being kind) came on covered in yellow feathers and performed a 'chicken dance'. How we had to control ourselves! After this, some of the mothers performed 'The Dance of the Seven Veils'. Most of them were quite large too. We had nothing but admiration for them but we were practically hysterical by then. Ah, but they were good times.

"I also recall the Annual Anglo-Argentine Society Barbecue at Sutton Valance Rugby Club. We had wonderful food, whole roasted lambs and *empanadas*. After the barbecue we all played games, rounders and so on. It was great fun.

"We were both on the Parent Teachers Association at St Teresa's School, and I can remember us running stalls at the annual school fetes. Sarah and Louise always helped us. At one of the school Sports Days I remember Sarah winning a sack race.

"Do you remember Bruce buying you a kaftan from a stall in London? I really liked it and he very kindly bought one for me, and guess what, I still have it! You lined the hood of yours – you were pretty good with the needle.

"I used to hire a hall for my daughters' birthday party. Sarah was very good at all the games and won quite a number of the prizes."

Frances Turner added to her recollections that Sarah always wore a bright yellow mac and hat, which made her look great.

Val adds: "Auntie Frances would tick the children off on the daily walk to school if they complained when it was raining. She'd say, 'Now, children, don't make a fuss. A little bit of rain never hurt anybody' even if it was thundering down, with the rain dripping off our noses!

"The children always went to each other's birthday parties. Another memory is of of Sarah saying to me as we were crossing Magazine Road – or trying to – 'Go on, Mummy, stop the traffic', because I would go to the middle of the road and hold up my hand to stop the cars so the children could cross."

Sheila Whitelegg was a babysitter for Sarah and Mark during the early Altrincham days. She remembers that the television was never on. The conversation was so lively and so stimulating that no diversions were required. There was always the background noise of the pet hamster on his wheel!

Another Ashford neighbour, **Tessa Flood**, remembers Sarah as bright and intelligent, organising her son Simon and Mark Hotter and their games. One afternoon Sarah kept the boys quiet for ages by reading stories. Tessa recalls Sarah's beautiful red hair, and watching 'The Magic Roundabout' at birthday parties. Sarah was so obedient and would help to manage the other little children.

Norman and Beth (Auntie Beff) Crump were the Hotters' next-door-neighbours-but-one in Ashford. Between them lived Max and Audrey Livesey. The three families shared many good moments together.

Beth recalls Sarah standing patiently waiting while her father Bruce, Max and Norman "were yakking on and on". Sarah, who had been sent to tell the men it was coffee time, went to Audrey to borrow the bell "'cos that's what Mummy does when she wants Daddy when he's out in the garden".

When Sarah and Mark went to visit Norman and Beth she always offered to help in some way, and would happily sit down with a blank sheet of paper and a box of crayons and produce a picture *(see below)*.

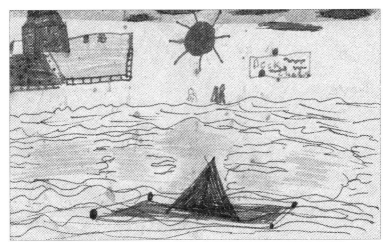

Norman tried to tease Sarah by calling her 'Sarah Jane', long after she had stamped her foot at him and emphasised "My name's Sarah LOUISE – not Sarah Jane!"

Beth recalls: "She was such a delight, with her lovely auburn hair, and tried to keep Mark in his place by scolding him if he outstepped the mark in her estimation. She was never precocious in her childhood years and was a lucky girl to have had such a loving Mum and Dad and a wide circle of friends and relations."

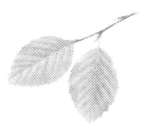

Chapter 3
LORETO
1975 – 1984

Knowledge is always accompanied with accessories
of emotion and purpose

A. N. Whitehead, Adventures of Ideas, 1933

IN August 1975 the Hotter family moved to Hale, about eight miles south of Manchester. Bruce had been moved as part of Barclay's reorganisation. He became Deputy Manager of the company's computer centre at Wythenshawe. The second house they viewed appealed to them immediately and they decided to buy it. Val still lives there now, enjoying her home and garden.

When nine-year-old Sarah was told of the imminent move to Cheshire she sat on the settee in Ashford with tears rolling down her face. Where was Cheshire? Was English spoken there?

If English was not spoken, this would be a horrendous problem for such a chatterbox. The silent tears were a strong signal; a rebuke, perhaps? A Sarah full of loud objection was one thing; a quiet miserable Sarah was a different kettle of fish!

When the Hotters visited St Vincent's Infant and Junior Schools in Altrincham in the summer before their move north, Mark refused to get out of the car to inspect his new school. There was no way he was going to investigate, and he sat scowling determinedly in the back seat, impervious to his parents' cheerful encouragement.

The date of the move, 1 August, was Bruce's birthday. Val bought presents for Sarah and Mark to give him. Early in the morning, all excited, they came banging on their parents' bedroom door. "Bloody kids! Go away!" was the immediate reaction. Then, hearing "Happy Birthday To You!" and realising the significance of the occasion, Bruce let them in.

Sarah and Mark were fascinated by the new house in Hale, and would chase about excitedly, investigating, exploring and rushing in to report new happenings. One of the things that particularly interested them was the house bell system, whereby a bell in each of the main rooms was connected to a pulley system in the kitchen with the appropriate room indicator 'waggling' when the bell was pressed. Soon after arriving Sarah and Mark were clumping up and down the stairs with their friends, testing each individual bell. The house had no carpets at the time and the place reverberated with the noise. The children would say, just as Val was on her way to the front door thinking a visitor had come: "Don't worry, Mummy, it's just us!"

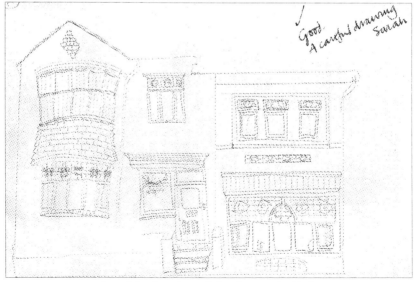

Sarah's drawing of the house in Hale

In the new house there were also Easter Egg Hunts. The house lent itself beautifully to long and exhausting hunts, since it had a cellar, two floors and an attic room. The clues were most unkindly spaced out, and the little ones would rush up and down the stairs. Sarah got most of the clues before Mark did, and she would have to be asked to stop so her little brother could have a go too.

A favourite occasion was the dressing-up Halloween party at the end of October, always held in the suitably mysterious cellar. The atmosphere with subdued lights and weird costumes was always quite hilarious. As Sarah and Mark became older and somewhat more sophisticated there were disco parties in the sitting room. On one occasion the disco party ended with a game of Murder in the Dark, a lovely amalgam of childhood and emerging sophistication.

On Sarah's 30th birthday party, held at a pub in Altrincham, Val offered to make a celebration cake, thinking in terms of the traditional fruit cake with white icing and posh squiggles. However, what Sarah most wanted was the famous 'Brown' chocolate cake, and that is what Val made. When Sarah's school friends saw the cakes they all exclaimed: "Oh, girls, LOOOK, Mrs Hotter's chocolate cake!"

Sarah attended St Vincent's RC Junior School in Orchard Road, Altrincham. On the first day of Sarah being deposited in this strange place, the class teacher looked at the child, then the mother, and said: "Don't worry; they all look scared when they first start."

Sarah's brother Mark was in the Infant Department. Sarah spent two years there, then passed the 11-plus examination, ready for the next stage of her education.

Loreto Convent Grammar School has existed in Altrincham since 1911 in premises which were once a doctor's house. Its reputation and its premises have grown steadily since, and there are now about eight hundred pupils, all girls. The Head Teacher, Sister Patricia Goodstadt, kindly set time aside for Val and me to visit the school and talk about Sarah with her and with Sarah's history teacher, Mrs Frances McGee.

I had no trouble finding the school. Just across the leafy main road from Manchester to Chester which runs across the front of the school is the spot where my Dad and I used to sit together to watch the cars go by in the years just after the war. In the late 1940s the cars had greater aesthetic appeal – Lagondas I especially liked – and there were far fewer of them, allowing time for contemplation as they passed slowly by. I remember sending models of these cars on my own imagined journeys as I played with my Dinkys at my home near Loreto School.

Thirty years later, when Sarah began her time at Loreto, that road to Chester – Dunham Road – had become a main feeder road

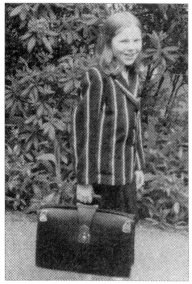

One of the 'wasps'!
September 1987.

for the M6 motorway. A footbridge had to be constructed so that the Loreto pupils, and the boys from neighbouring North Cestrian Grammar School, could cross safely.

One morning in September 1977, Val and Sarah approached the footbridge on Sarah's first day at Loreto. But they were not to cross it together. "This is far enough," announced Sarah. Val was dismissed and Sarah entered her new school as she wished, unaccompanied, in her uniform of navy, maroon and cream striped blazer, a matching tie, a navy cardigan edged at collar and cuffs with maroon and cream, a creamy yellow blouse, beige knee-length stockings, and regulation brown

shoes. Val thinks a collection of uniformed Loreto girls looked like a swarm of wasps. Val also remembers purchasing a regulation navy blue mackintosh which Sarah hardly ever wore, even in the rain.

Loreto Convent Grammar School has a reputation for academic excellence. The administrative offices are in what was once the doctor's house. The pupils, mostly but not all from Roman Catholic families, are drawn from the main towns of North Cheshire: Altrincham, Knutsford, Lymm, Warrington and Sale.

Sister Patricia Goodstadt, the Head Teacher of Loreto Convent Grammar School, is a member of the Institute of the Blessed Virgin Mary (IBVM). The Institute was founded by Mary Ward (1585 -1645), who was born into a Yorkshire family which upheld the Catholic faith through a long period of persecution in the England of that time. Mary Ward became a nun, but having declared to her Superiors "the exceeding difficulty which I found in embracing that vocation", she established in 1609 at St Omer in northern France a boarding school for English girls and a day school for the children of

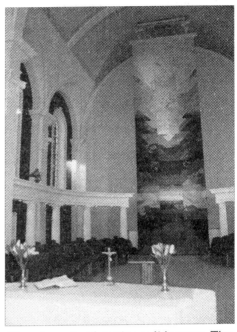

The chapel at Loreto as it is now. The tapestry is by Maureen Kelly. It has changed since Sarah's days.

the town. Subsequently, she opened many schools in different cities, to provide a new type of religious life for women, dedicated to the education of Catholic girls.

The educational philosophy of the Loreto schools is based on the Gospel values of Freedom, Justice, Sincerity, Truth and Joy, which were the core values of Margaret Ward and are the guiding principles of the schools today. All Loreto students are encouraged to be "seekers of truth and doers of justice", just as Mary Ward asked of her pupils four hundred years ago.

When I visited Loreto school with Val I was immediately aware of a warm relaxed atmosphere. I had been told to expect some merriment, as well as academic insights, when we met Sister Patricia and Frances McGee. A 'Meeting in Progress; Do Not Disturb' notice was hung on the door. Coffee and biscuits were produced and we had a joyful conversation about Sarah, liberally

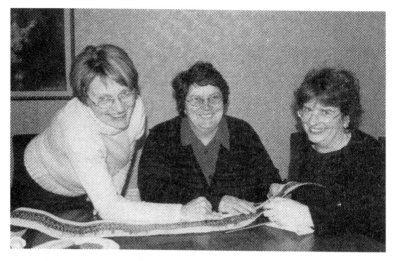

*Sister Patricia (centre) pictured with Frances McGee (right)
and Val Hotter (left).*

dotted with amusing asides that underlined Sister Patricia's philosophy – very evident in Loreto School – that "if life isn't fun, real
learning is not happening". To emphasise this point, Sister
Patricia said: "People who don't believe this don't live at Loreto."
Sister Patricia and her deputy, Frances McGee, are people who
have a twinkle in the eye but don't miss a trick. Our time together had echoes of that first time I met Sarah in my office at Beeston.

Sister Patricia produced some of Sarah's school records. There
was the admission form for Sarah Louise Hotter, September 1977,
signed by her father. There appears to be some uncertainty about
the date of her birth; 1965 had been changed to 1966 in a way that
suggests either date might apply! Sarah had been baptised and
had made her First Communion. There were no particular health
problems.

It was clear at once that Loreto School remembers Sarah Hotter
with admiration. Frances McGee was the history teacher from
Sarah's Year 10, when Sarah was 15. The class was in a prefabri-
cated building, and twenty one years later Mrs McGee can
remember exactly where each pupil sat for her lessons; it was one
of those classes which establishes a particularly strong rapport

with the teacher. Sarah sat on the left, at the front. Mrs McGee recalls Sarah's immediate and astute grasp of all the concepts and insights of history, and her active involvement with the subject. She was very well read. She was interested in the different cultures and periods of history, and how people lived. "Everything was very easy about Sarah," says Mrs McGee. "Her work was easy to mark, so well presented, and never handed in late. She was intellectually challenging, and outpaced me."

Mrs McGee took Sarah on to A-level, where she studied the history of Britain in the nineteenth century, from the Prime Ministership of Lord Liverpool, 1812, to the outbreak of the First World War in 1914. With another teacher, Mr Stanley, Sarah studied the history of Europe, with special attention to Germany and Russia, from the late nineteenth to the twentieth century.

Most of the ablest Loreto girls applied to one of the Oxford colleges, and it had long been evident that Sarah would be in this category. Mrs McGee prepared her accordingly.

Lively as she was in her history lessons, and versatile as she

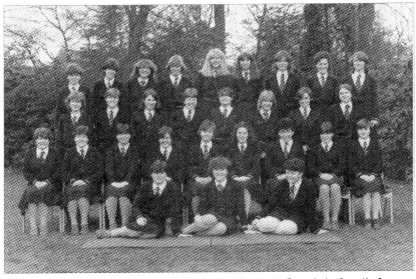

The Fifth Form (5W) at Loreto in April 1982. Sarah is fourth from the left in the second row down, standing behind the seated girls.

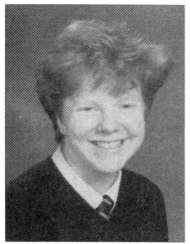

Sarah as a Sixth-former

was in her grasp of other subjects, Sarah is remembered as "very quiet in many ways". She was very well behaved; not sporty. She worked hard and methodically. Val recalls Sarah at her books in the early morning during the weekends, particularly before exams, and entreating her, "Don't worry, you'll be fine."

Sarah sang in the Loreto School Choir, but was not a principal performer. As a Third Year pupil she took part in a Sixth Form drama production. She did not enjoy performing all that much, but would do well if asked. She took part in school Gilbert and Sullivan productions, and in the play 'Poverty Knock' performed by the Loreto pupils at Quarry Bank Mill, Styal. The manager of the Mill had attended the performance at school, and invited the production to come to the Mill.

Other characters in her "powerful, occasionally wild" year group were more to the fore. Sarah was always involved in the life of the school; Sister Patricia noted her positive contribution to the ethos of Loreto. Sarah had "a kind of shyness"; she accepted her fine mind but never bragged about it. She was on the school's Pupils Committee but did not seek the position of Head Girl. In a school photograph of a small group of Sixth Form girls, her teachers see her as "really engaging the camera, yet keeping herself to herself". Sister Patricia and Mrs McGee have no doubt that Sarah was happy at school.

Sarah's A-level subjects were History, Chemistry, English and General Studies. She gained 'A' grades in all of them, proving herself a versatile as well as able pupil. Sarah applied to three of the colleges at Oxford University. Bruce accompanied her by train to her interview at Jesus College. She had applied to two women-only colleges at Oxford, but decided Jesus was the one for her. She told Val and Bruce that she would accept an offer from Jesus, but not from the two other colleges. Val is still bemused by the thought of turning down a place at any Oxford college!

Sarah had also applied to Bristol University, who invited her for interview. She would travel down by train. Val and Sarah arranged to meet outside Loreto on the appointed day, for Val to drive Sarah to the station. At the agreed time, Sarah was waiting with her bag and some books, looking nonchalant. Val handed Sarah a telegram from Jesus College that had come that morning. It stated, rather cryptically: "Elected to Open Exhibition. Letter follows. Jesus College". Val was not exactly sure what the message meant. Sarah was! As soon as she read it, her books flew up in the air and landed all over the path. She dashed back to school and into Sister Patricia's office. Val remembers being left "a hundred yards behind". She recalls Sister Patricia emerging from her office, "pink and totally delighted". Val explained that she was there to set Sarah on her way to Bristol but Sister Patricia suggested a phone call to Bristol to say that Sarah would not now be attending.

So Sarah and Val made the much shorter journey home to Hale. Bruce was phoned at work, and in Val's words "all was wonderful". Family friends Liz and Clive arrived with a bottle of champagne. The Barclay's Bank Computer Centre was now based at Radbroke Hall near Knutsford. A colleague of Bruce recalls vividly the day when Sarah's success became known. "We were sharing offices in the Open Plan Section, Block 10, right next to each other, and he was bursting to tell me the news. I don't think there was a happier or a prouder man in the whole of Cheshire that day."

DUNE SLIDING, CAMPING, INTER-RAILING AND SCRUMPTIOUS FOOD!
Some of Sarah's early travels

Sarah was a great traveller. From dune-sliding as a baby, to the far south of Argentina, the wanderlust was there. When the family bought their first car, a Morris 1000 – Sarah was about two at this time – many happy hours were spent on the Camber Sands or the Romney Marsh area in Kent. Wherever there were sand dunes, Bruce, Valerie and Sarah would sit on the top, looking out at the sea. Sarah would promptly start shuffling down to the bottom of the dune. Bruce or Valerie would pick her up, place her on the top, and she would immediately shuffle down to the bottom again. Sarah didn't walk till she was twenty months old as she progressed so efficiently by shuffling on her bottom everywhere. Many strong material 'cast iron' pants were made for her, and she shuffled them all out in a matter of days!

There were visits to Buenos Aires to the family in Argentina. In Sarah's journal for one visit to Buenos Aires at Christmas 1988 are the words: "When anyone asks me what we did the first day in BA, they'll not believe the answer. We did a mini-tour of the cemeteries. There were some English bulbs to plant in a family grave in the British Cemetery so we piled into the somewhat battered car and off we went. We had to stifle giggles at the people coming into the graveyard clutching great bunches of rather weary gladioli. Then we noticed that the crypts had little tin chimneys sticking out of the top. Daddy commented that maybe it was so the corpses could breathe. And that was it... the Brown cackle of Maureen, Mummy and I was heard to ring out across the graveyard. Speculating on the real purpose of the chimneys only made us worse, as gruesome visions came to mind.

"So we were not in the calmest of moods to face Teddy's next stop on the tour, the Chacarita. This was a great cemetery next door, the largest urban cemetery in the world. It was filled with palatial crypts, marble monuments with small chapels inside, great gold crosses and elaborate lace tablecloths, statues of women with faces cast down, and other figures in great draperies.

"Daddy didn't want to be there at all and the women were in an advanced state of hysteria. But Teddy was intent on showing us the tomb of Juan Peron, which was guarded by suitably fierce-looking *policia*. Teddy threatened to get out and inform them that we were British tourists and the image of us waving Union Jacks and singing 'The Falklands are British' was enough to keep the hysteria bubbling. From there we went to the places where the poor came to rest. There were makeshift wooden crosses above the graves, which would be emptied if the payments were not kept up. As we drove out of the cemetery we met a cortege of

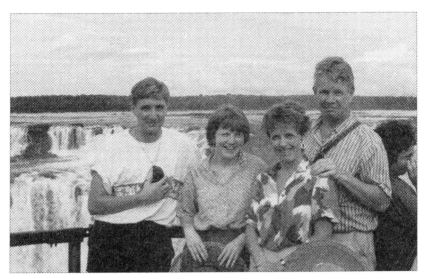

The Hotter family at Iguazu Falls in Argentina, 1988

about ten black cars. I just hid my face as I couldn't stop laughing. OK if we had a car crash, though, quipped Teddy – not far to go with the bodies. By this time Daddy was looking somewhat green, but I haven't had such a laugh for a very long time ."

On one of the trips to her aunt and uncle in Vancouver, sixteen year old Sarah – this time on her own – was taken on a camping trip into the Rocky Mountains. On the trip eastwards towards the Rockies, Sarah says: "We drove on almost to Banff, and as we entered the area we saw a huge mountain that looked like a cliff rising out of the trees. We stopped at a viewpoint to look at another amazing mountain which resembled a wave with the crest about to curl over. On the plaque was a very true quotation: 'Never before did I behold such a perfect resemblance to the waves of the ocean. When looking upon them the imagination is apt to say, these once must have been liquid.'"

Sarah was introduced to lovely places and different foods. She notes: "I had lobster Bisque soup (so-so) with still warm bread, followed by Salmon Wellington with courgettes and rice, followed by choc ice cream – SCRUMPTIOUS (not quite up Mark's street, though), then with a friend a breakfast of blueberry hot-cakes with blueberry sauce."

Sarah did a few Inter-Rail trips round Europe. One of them entailed a journey from London to Naples via Strasbourg, where her pen-friend Martine lives. In Strasbourg, made warmly welcome by Martine's family and their dog, Sarah tasted the traditional *Choucroute Alsacienne*, creamy white cabbage with pork and sausages, to which you add salt, onion, bay and cream, and eat with potato. There were also the famous Alsacienne *Backeofe* and *Tarte Flambée*. Sarah records on one occasion: "For dinner (major events of the day, meals!) artichoke, palm hearts and asparagus salads. A breakfast of chocolate and vanilla cake and coffee. The most scrumptious lunch ever: trout with almonds, then exotic fruit salad. Dinner was pancakes with cheese and mushroom, followed by *crème caramel*.

"From Strasbourg to Rome; after the mountains, acres of vineyards, sunflowers and maize. Arrived in Rome, managed to get seats on an 'every second lamp post' train to Naples, where we went for a meal at a local restaurant; spaghetti with oil and garlic and the inevitable *acqua minerale*, then to a *gelateria* for a real *gelato limone* – yum! Gorgeous breakfast at local café, *cappuccino* coffee and *croissants*. We had breakfast at the youth hostel once but the coffee was so foul we treated ourselves to breakfast out. On other days we had custard cream *croissants* and delicious doughnuts. We passed through a town called Positano which had cream and peach buildings literally grasping the mountainside."

Sarah had a strategy in Italy with chat-up pests:

> • *Ignore them*
> • *Pretend to understand every word they say but refuse to speak Italian so they can't make remarks about you*
> • *Tell them you're Russian – they've no hope of speaking the language*
> • *When you have to speak to each other, eg on train when surrounded by about five blokes on the uptake, speak French or English with a strong accent!*

Yet often when they left, the 'pests' would shake Sarah's hand and say *Ciao*, as formal as can be!

Rome had the most scrumptious ice cream – chocolate chips in chocolate ice cream, made into a cake, covered in chocolate chips and cream and eaten off a little silver paper plate.

Also in Rome, the local traffic scene – "absolute mayhem outside our window" – dogs, cars, people, buses, taxis and above all, scooters, barely missing each other and all blaring their horns.

Sarah changed into promenade gear and to cries of *"Alo"* and *"Speek Inglis"* got some takeaway pizza and freshly roasted peanuts, followed by a Martini. This latter was accompanied by a very persistent chat-up from two blokes. Moral of the day – when a male asks you if a seat is free, say NO!

"A small town in France. The meal was amazing; tomato soup, a Swedish dish with anchovies, rice, vegetables, Dauphin potatoes, salads, fruit salad, cheese and bread. Much too much food, after which we sat outside with dogs, stars and moon."

In Barcelona "we sat on a bench opposite a group of old men who were fantastic entertainment. One or two solidly kept their places but the rest were constantly moving from bench to bench, sitting or leaning on the back. As voices rose, one or other of the men would stand, hitch his belt aggressively and make as if to leave, but with a few words he'd be smiling, at himself as much as anything, then he'd hitch his trousers in a way that meant he was smoothing down his feathers so he could sit down again. One disagreement got to the point where one chap plonked himself on our bench, casting disgusted

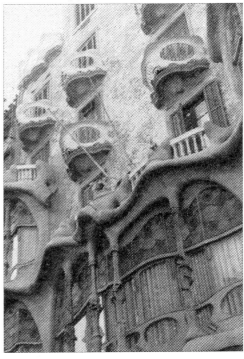

A snapshot from Barcelona

looks across the way – perhaps someone had insulted his friend in the wheelchair; who knows?

"Then another coffee, a different café. And we watch a little girl amuse herself by using the drinking fountain as a tool for spraying everyone in sight and creating a lovely damp patch so that all the lads on their BMXs come to skiddy crunches with the floor. The square has an odd mixture of people, backpackers, tourists, trendies, old chaps, families and kids, and the rather squalid end of the scale as well, drunks and 'street bums.'"

From Barcelona to Granada: "The scenery was gorgeous. A wonderful harvest moon reflecting on a calm sea. We were continually going through short tunnels as the tracks passed through the hills that came down to the sea. We could see the lights of cars as they wound round the coast road. Below on the long sandy beaches there were fisherman with their lights beside them. We

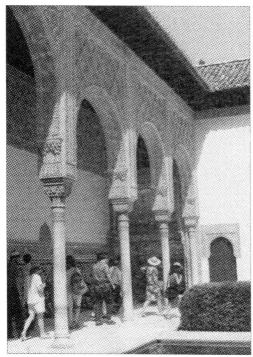

Granada: the Alhambra

passed through several towns where everyone was out on the streets or on their balconies finishing dinner. We could hear the crickets and smell the rich colour of the trees and shrubs. But we had to go to bed on our top couchettes because the other two passengers had switched the light off by twelve."

Sarah read a wall plaque in Alhambra, Granada, which said: "Give him alms, woman, because there is nothing, nothing so sad as to be blind in Granada."

In Tarragona "the food was great in quality

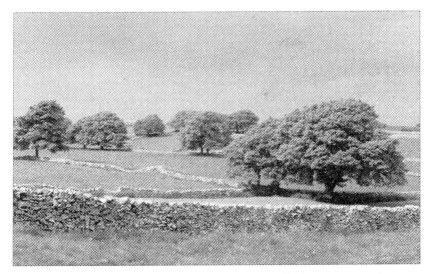

Sarah loved the Derbyshire Dales

and quantity. All for the kingly sum of about £3.50 there was *gaspacho*, salads, mussels, squid, quiches, then *paella*, chicken, and a sort of haggis boiled together with veg. In a pan, stuffed squid, stuffed aubergine, then the buffet of desserts – *crème caramel*, *Crema Catalunya*, rice pudding, melons, a cake."

The Hotters had happy times visiting the Derbyshire Dales and the Lake District and both these areas were well loved by Sarah. The favourite section of the Lakes was the north west, particularly the Cockermouth area, which became quite special. Once Sarah started working in London she missed the hills and would often return, to have some lovely walks and take in the fresh air. She loved coming back to the Manchester area because she knew she would be near the hills. The Hotters would just don their heavy weather clothing and trudge off.

A NICE PLACE FOR LUNCH
Caron (Leech) Walker, a friend from school days, recalls some journeys with Sarah:

"Sarah's journey was not only about living life to its fullest, but also about laughter. In 1988 we visited Istanbul and parts of west-

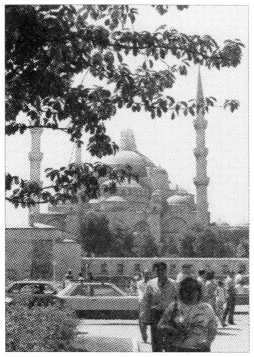
Turkey - the Blue Mosque

ern Turkey together and for years we have giggled helplessly at the memories of those days.

"I remember an early morning walk through the meandering streets as we followed the hotel receptionist in search of a health centre. Sarah had a severe attack of sunstroke and the receptionist delivered us safely to a doctor. The doctor proceeded to interview a sales rep as Sarah lay on the couch before finally, whilst muttering under her breath about foolish tourists, wearily dishing out some cream and tablets. The irony of the tale was that in those days of short skirts and skimpy bikinis, Sarah and I walked the streets of Istanbul looking like a pair of Victorian schoolmistresses, Sarah because she feared the sun's effects and myself because I was overcompensating for local sensitivities as I dragged Sarah from one vitally important mosque to another. She, of course, cheerily threw herself into each new experience with awesome energy.

"I also remember the lazy Sunday mornings spent over newspapers and coffee as we deconstructed the problems of British society, solved the Kashmiri problem or redrew the map of Europe, convinced that if only the politicians would leave things to us, we would beat the lot of them! Then we would clear away, wash up, and leave the world's problems to another day as we sought out a nice place for lunch!"

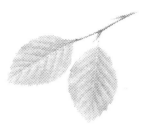

Chapter 4
OXFORD
1984 – 1987

Make your friends your teachers and mingle the pleasures
of conversation with the advantages of instruction

Baltasar Gracian, The Art of Worldly Wisdom, 1647

Anne (Fletcher) Teckman became a friend of Sarah's at Oxford. She writes:
"We went up to Jesus College on 10 October 1984. None of the freshers (new students) had met before and because we all came from varied backgrounds, different parts of the country, and with different expectations, it was a nerve-wracking time. I moved into Staircase III Room 10, a girls-only staircase. That day I met my next door neighbour, Sarah. I am sure most people were terrified! I certainly imagined everyone would be cleverer and more exciting than me. Sarah admitted later that she had felt the same but decided on arrival to give a completely opposite impression. Sarah walked into my room in wide-legged trousers, shirt, tie and trilby! She looked incredibly cool and trendy and I was very impressed.

"I soon found out that Sarah was nothing like her first, rather intimidating, impression. She proved to be a gentle, funny, intelligent and warm friend. Sarah and I had more in common than just our red hair. We had both been accepted to read Modern History

31

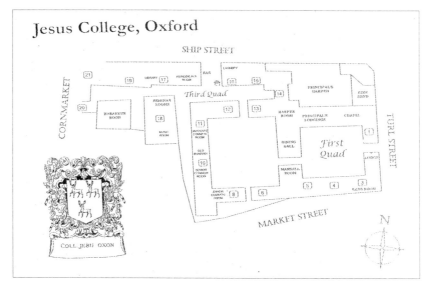

The layout of Jesus College, Oxford

and we held the two Exhibitions awarded that year. Exhibitions are traditional bursaries offered to students, Scholarships being more valuable. Historically, Exhibitions had finance attached to them to help with students' living costs; now, they are used just to recognise academic achievement. They are awarded on entry to the university and can be withdrawn. Sarah and I both managed to keep ours for three years.

"There were eight historians accepted by Jesus in 1984; Sarah, me, Rufus, Rob, Heledd, Rachel, Trevelyan and Rosie. We all became good friends, particularly Sarah, Rufus, Rob, Rosie and me. Sarah was a good student. She worked hard and gained excellent results. She was popular not only with the other history students but also with her tutors. Sarah and I shared a Scout. Scouts were the college servants responsible for cleaning our rooms and staircases. Ours was called Ray. He came every morning. In addition to cleaning, he made our beds and washed up for us. Sarah and I were both so embarrassed about this, and used to hide our mugs and plates in our desk drawers. Inevitably, Ray always found them! He must have thought we were very funny and always gave us extra pudding when he was serving in Hall.

"Sarah got very involved in music at College, becoming a member of the Choir. She was also a very keen rower. We went to an event laid on for Freshers by the different groups at College, and decided to have a go at rowing. Sarah rowed on Bow Side and I on Stroke. We had to train very hard, cycling or running down to the river on training days to be there for 6.30am. Sarah excelled, and made it into the Jesus women's' First Eight crew. This meant that she rowed against other Colleges at Eights (summer) and Torpids (Spring), and got to wear the lovely bright green College vest!

"We spent much of our free time putting the world to rights, either in the College bar or outside in the quad. I remember that during our first week Sarah and I stayed up all night talking, and then went straight to a Tutorial. It was the first time that either of us had stayed up all night and we thought we were very grown up!

"The college bar was a natural focus of college life but I remember that Sarah did try to drag us up to a more sophisticated level. Typical of this was the night when she and her flatmates (in her second year at Oxford Sarah shared a flat with two others) held a cocktail party.

"The trio invested

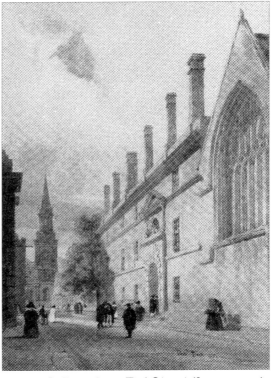

Jesus College from Turl Street (from a postcard published by The Isis Press)

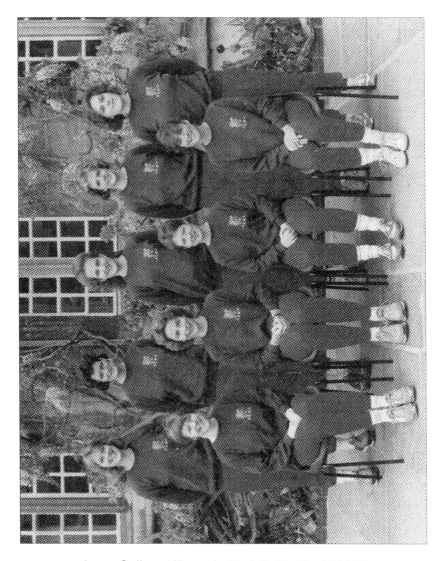

Jesus College Women's First Eight, Torpid 1987.
L-R (back row), Anna Bean, Katherine William-Powlett, Harriet
Hepburn, Mary Nottidge, Anne Bevitt; front row, Sarah Hotter,
Louise Marchant (captain), Lisa Mellor (cox), Jennie Kassanoff.
(Photo: Gillman and Soame, 8 St Michael's Street, Oxford)

in cocktail shakers, glasses and all the ingredients needed for a modest array of concoctions. As usual Sarah looked great, wearing vintage clothes before they were fashionable. Sarah was a regular attender at Mahogany, the hairdressers near the college. She offered herself as a model to hairdressing trainees, and unlike anyone else, let them do whatever they wanted! She frequently returned with dramatically coloured highlights in her hair, and strange cuts, but she always had the style to carry it off.

"Sarah and I also went to our first Ball together. It was at Exeter College in March 1985. We went

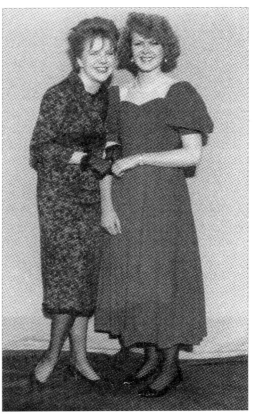

Two redheads ready for the Ball

with a small group of friends, some from college, some from home, and enjoyed an evening of great music and dancing. Sarah wore a fantastic turquoise and black suit (vintage again, I think).

"Our gang was reunited again in the summer of 1998. We all went to the Jesus College Gaudy, a get-together for the college graduates where three or so year-groups are invited back for a Dinner. Our year, 1984, attended with a year from the '60s and one from the '20s. We spent the weekend in Oxford and on the Sunday Sarah and I took a walk by the river. It was there that she told me she had a brain tumour. I was very shocked but also very moved by how strong and brave she was in the telling. This was the last time I saw Sarah.

"We kept in touch by phone and I was reminded again how incredibly brave and strong Sarah was when we spoke early in 1999. My Dad died suddenly in January of that year and because Sarah had lost her father too, I had an overwhelming urge to call her and talk about it. But because of her prognosis I didn't want to talk to her about such a gloomy subject. So I called her and in the course of the chat I told Sarah about my Dad, intending to pass quickly on to something else. Sarah, being Sarah, wouldn't let me – she said, 'Go on, tell me all about it, what happened... ' That was my final conversation with Sarah."

THE TIGER EFFECT
Rosie Edge, a friend of Sarah's at Jesus College, writes:
"How can you explain a friendship? The facts are easy to explain, the feelings less so. Sarah and I were friends for fifteen years. In that time there were periods when we saw each other every day, didn't communicate for months, kept in touch by post-card or had the occasional meal out. Each time we picked up as we left off, without too much effort.

"So, of fifteen years, what stands out for me? My initial memory of is Sarah with short spiky hair, in pink dungarees and bright red lipstick. She once told me that arriving at Oxford was quite daunting and that dressing for confidence was her way of coping. I also remember the time she got her hair, still spiky and short at this point, dyed with flecks of blond and black. The effect was like a tiger – fantastic! The whole time I knew her, Sarah always struck me as a very well-groomed person, nails always beautifully kept, hair always well cut, even during her shaggy dog look!

"What else then? Well, her energy and enthusiasm of course, from making costumes for college plays, to singing in the Oxford Bach Choir and Jesus College Choir, to rowing, to history, to teaching, to working. Example; we shared a terrifying tutor (who shall remain nameless) and my only comfort was that Sarah was there for moral support. We even went on a day trip to Dorchester Abbey together in an effort to enthuse ourselves – more for the tea and cakes in the Cathedral coffee shop than for any other reason, I suspect.

"Other things; endless cups of tea in Jesus quad, civilised din-

36

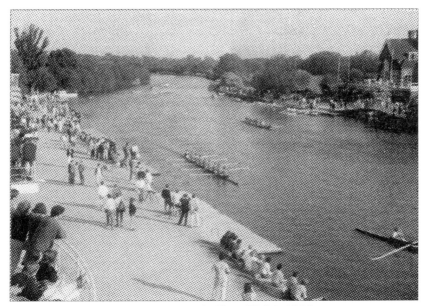

Jesus' women's First Eight, 1985

ner parties in London, wandering around Santiago de Compostela in the sunshine, the way Sarah's eyes crinkled up when she laughed, standing in a field of oilseed rape with Anne Fletcher – red hair and yellow flowers.

"What I'm doing now is due a great deal to Sarah's inspiration. I was very envious when she gave up her job to go travelling round South America with Mark. It was somewhere I'd always wanted to go but I didn't have the guts to do what she did. It took me a lot longer to do something similar, and talking to her inspired me a lot to have the courage to change.

"So it was that I left for Spain just at the point when Sarah was becoming more ill. Every day I feel that I am following her example and getting on with life, and that's the most significant memory anyone could have."

THE CHOIR AND THE BUMPS
Val Hotter recalls a visit to Sarah at Oxford:
"Everyone has a clear memory of a beautiful day or a beautiful

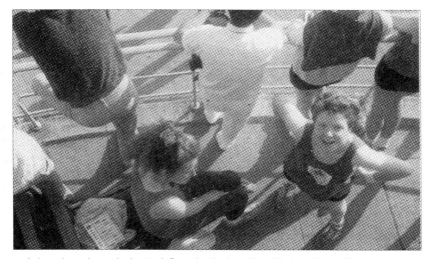

A lovely relaxed shot of Sarah during the Eights Boat Race, 1985

occasion. One of my loveliest memories is the day I spent in Oxford with Sarah in 1987, her final year at Jesus College.

"She was rowing in the college women's' First Eight, and the day coincided with an evening performance of her singing with the Oxford Bach Choir in a performance of Bach's B Minor Mass, a wonderful oratorio.

"Bruce and Mark had been unable to join us so I went to Oxford on my own. When I arrived there was a note pinned to the door of Sarah's flat, to tell me where she was. I made my way down to the river and it was a magic scene – a lovely warm sunny June day, people sitting in chairs or on the grass in friendship, quite a few of them with drinks in hand, enjoying the lovely atmosphere and looking forward to the rowing. I joined them, and although not entirely au fait with the intricacies of rowing and the 'Bumps', I was aware of Sarah and her companions doing their enthusiastic and level best to win.

"Some time during the afternoon Sarah had to return to the Sheldonian Theatre for the choir rehearsal. I clearly remember sitting high up in the Theatre enjoying every minute. When it got to the opening bars of the Gloria – a stirring, wonderful piece of music – she looked up at me and grinned broadly: she knew how

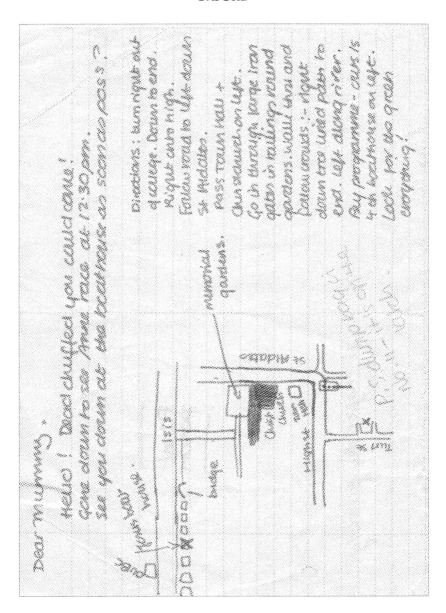

Sarah's note to her mother, pinned on the door of her flat, 1987

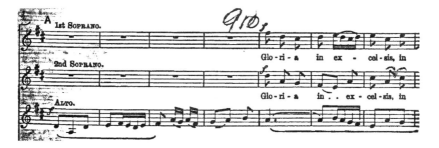

A shared moment as the choir sang the opening bars of the "Gloria"

I would have been enjoying it. I grinned back; a lovely shared moment.

"We then returned to the river for the finals of the Bumps, after which Sarah, together with some of the others, was picked up by some of the lads and dumped unceremoniously into the river, with everyone clapping and cheering. In the evening I sat again in the Sheldonian listening to the wonderful music – a glorious day, full of music, fun and sunshine."

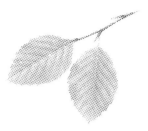

Chapter 5
LONDON
1987 – 1991

We cannot remain consistent with the world
save by growing inconsistent with our past selves

Havelock Ellis, The Dance of Life, 1923

IN the summer of 1987 Val, Bruce and Mark Hotter attended Sarah's graduation ceremony in the Sheldonian Theatre at Oxford University. In ten written papers taken in her Final Examinations, Sarah gained a good Honours degree (2:1) in History. By this time, she had been interviewed by three companies. Later that year Sarah began work with International Computers Limited (ICL) at their Finsbury Park offices in London. She was employed in a small team selling computerised information systems to the legal profession.

I travelled to London to meet four of Sarah's former colleagues at ICL. They were Chris Brandt, Miranda Freeman, Andy Long and Maxine Vaughan.

Our meeting place was well chosen, a quiet cosy Nepalese restaurant just two minutes' walk from Euston Station. I wasn't to know that my train from Crewe would depart almost an hour late, full of Spanish football fans singing and celebrating Real Madrid's defeat of Bayer Leverkusen the previous evening in Glasgow in the final of the European Champions Cup. OLE! OLE! It occurred

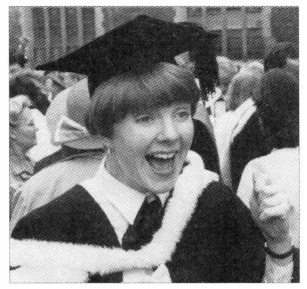

Sarah's graduation day, 21 May 1988

to me that Sarah would be amused by this!

In London Chris, Miranda, Andy, Maxine and I chatted over poppadums, ricy spicy savouries and Cobra Indian beer. Chris recalled a visit to Twickenham rugby ground in 1989 to watch England play the Pumas, an Argentinian side. "Whereas we all looked as if we had just got out of bed," said Chris, "Sarah dressed for the occasion, in an outfit of emerald green velvet, with an equally striking hat on her orange-red hair; she looked really striking, and lots of heads turned."

Bill Rodwell, another former colleague at ICL, also remembers that occasion. "During those happy far-off days of ICL, I arranged for a party of about fifteen people to watch the England v Argentina rugby match at Twickenham. Included in the party were three ladies: Sarah Hotter's mother (who hailed from Argentina), Sarah herself and Isabel Botilho, an attractive euro-grad on secondment from ICL in Lisbon. We all had a couple of drinks before the game and set off for Twickenham to take our seats in the East Stand. The visiting Argentinian team came out first, followed by the home English team. I happened to notice the reaction of Sarah and Isabel as the teams came out. They fairly obviously were transfixed by one of the English players, Jeremy Guscott, the England centre. I believe they watched Guscott for the rest of the game and were fairly oblivious to the activities of the other twenty nine players.

"For the record, England won comfortably. The most memorable moment in the whole game was when the Argentinian prop Frederico Mendes, who was then still a schoolboy, knocked out the 6ft 7in England second row forward Paul Ackford (then a Chief Inspector in the Metropolitan Police) with a tremendous right-hand punch. Paul Ackford was pole-axed. (Hello! Hello! Hello! What's going on here?)"

Chris was not sure if Sarah was sporty in the widest sense, but she did like rugby. Sarah's mother Val was also present at the Twickenham game, which took place just seven years after the Falklands War. Chris thinks Val was more affected than Sarah by the occasional anti-Argentina songs and comments from the crowd that day. Chris ascribes the comments more to beer than to hatred.

Chris had been to Argentina on business and in Buenos Aires he had met Maureen, Val's sister, and Maureen's husband Teddy. Chris noticed Sarah's involvement in her wider family. Sarah was a very family-orientated person, able to make and maintain close loving relationships. Moreover, she showed a keen interest, as genuine as it was unusual, in the families and concerns of her friends.

Maxine and Sarah would spend many Saturday evenings drinking wine in Maxine's flat. Their conversation centred on putting the world to rights – and eyeing up men! Sarah and Maxine had both been educated at religious foundations, with their associated rituals. They talked a lot about what they had sung at school, and for both of them choral music had been the main spiritual dimension of their education. It was an uplifting powerful experience, blended with what Maxine describes as "a weird feeling of calmness" for them to be in a choir that was performing in a big church or cathedral. Sarah was continually tra-la-ing or humming in her flat, which for Maxine could be a bit much by the end of a long weekend!

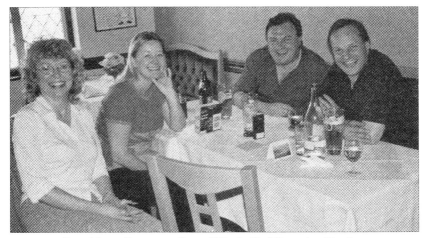

Sarah's colleagues from ICL. L-R: Miranda, Maxine, Andy and Chris.

Maxine remembers Sarah as a 'culture vulture' – she went to lots of plays, exhibitions and concerts.

For all their discussions about politics and religion, Maxine felt that at that time, in their early twenties, they had little real experience of life. Her colleagues knew Sarah was a Christian, they were less aware of her Catholic upbringing. They saw her as a socialist; she had "that Labour look, red like her hair"'. She was a *Guardian* reader because, she said, she liked the Arts section. Her other colleagues veered more towards the *Daily Mail*.

Sarah had clear views of her own, but apart from gentle ribbing, she never attacked views which differed from her own. She was seen as non-confrontational.

Miranda saw Sarah as a person who hid her light under a bushel. She was reticent about her achievements. Sarah was interesting, attractive, always fun, good for a chat and a laugh, yet "not out there on the London scene". But in spite of this reticence and apparent lack of confidence in herself during the ICL period, Sarah went on to success in two diverse careers, as a foreign language teacher and as a museum community and education officer.

Andy did not think that Sarah, with her interest in the underdog and her concern for the problems of people in underdeveloped countries, would stay long at ICL. The team saw Sarah as strikingly bright, but felt the corporate London 'big business' ambience caused her to try and conceal her cleverness. The London business scene can pressurise people to adopt an air of being glamorous, but the team felt Sarah's preference, out of working hours, would be to walk in the Dales with her family. Sarah was a down-to-earth person, for whom ICL was "too glitzy, too impersonal".

Commercial pressures coupled with the drive for profits, caused the ICL managers to try and exert more control over the teams. The managers, says Andy, lived for their work, competing among themselves for the biggest bonuses, whereas the legal team were "groovy", helped each other, and enjoyed life outside work. The legal team was in effect a separate company.

Sarah "loathed and hated office politics with a vengeance". She didn't smoke, but would join the smokers in their lairs during office breaks, to "catch up on the goss" and laugh about it. But ultimately, these dealings were of no interest to her.

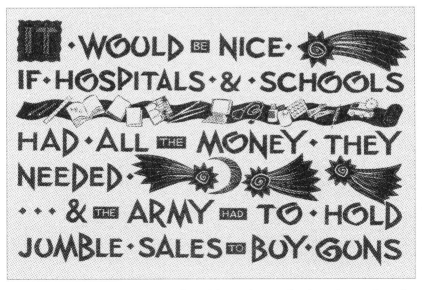

This was a favourite card of Sarah's and was displayed prominently in the kitchen at home (Design: Kate Charlesworth)

The team thought there was no question of Sarah remaining long in this situation; indeed, to them her long trip with Mark to South America was a major turning point in her life. Maxine, who remained in touch with Sarah, feels that it was only after South America with Mark that Sarah really "came into her own as a woman".

Until then, she thinks, and perhaps largely because of her years in a girls-only school and at Oxford, Sarah was not all that confident in herself; certainly not in male company. It was only in her last year at ICL, having made the decision to leave, that Sarah "opened up, and became much more confessional". Maxine was aware of Sarah's closeness to Mark; she thinks neither would have ventured to South America without the other, and to her, perhaps the real story of the trip was the bonding of Sarah and Mark.

Maxine says she would not normally stay in contact with the parents of her friends, but she feels she has inherited Sarah through Val. She misses Sarah very much. In the ICL days she and Sarah enjoyed visiting churches. They would light candles together. Maxine still does.

THE SALSA
Maxine Vaughan writes:

"One Sunday afternoon Sarah and I were mooching around the kitchen supping coffee in her apartment at Islington. It was an unimportant sort of day, neither of us was inclined to take advantage of the wealth of activities London was offering and work was looming for us Monday. Sarah and I met through work (ICL) in 1989 in the very gloomy and unglamorous surroundings of Feltham, Middlesex. Sarah and I had fallen for the concept of 'come work in the London bright lights, tall shiny buildings, endless Italian sandwich bars, suited men of the eligible variety'. But here we were in Feltham where the only bright light was the glare of the floodlights at the nearby Remand Centre.

"The day I first saw Sarah she was marching down a green linoleum corridor wielding a notepad. I remember the shock of red hair, the twinkling pair of eyes and the warm smile. Later she did tell me that the smile was because she knew I was the new girl and was probably suffering from location adjustment. We were

Mother's Day card
from Sarah to Val
in 1988
(Hallmark Cards;
Linus © 1952
United Feature
Syndicate Inc)

introduced shortly afterwards, and the rest is history...

"Now back to the Sunday in question... We were in the process of exploring our options in respect of exciting new things to do. For Sarah and me, the repertoire to this point had included theatre, movies, nightclubs and restaurants; the usual. We decided that we should cast our net wider in order to meet some nice young gentlemen. Sarah felt that we needed to do 'something active'. Suddenly a grin spread across her face and she raced out of the room. She reappeared brandishing a magazine. 'I've got it!' Flushed, she thumbed frantically through the pages. 'What? What?' I said. Sarah's concentration was total; no reply; then a small grunt, meaning 'Shhhh!' I was quiet.

"Then she let out a loud screech, and slapped the open magazine in front of me. It read: 'Come and Join Us and Learn the Salsa. Meet New People! Get into the Sensuous Rhythm of the Latins!'

"I gasped. Looking back, I see that Sarah was preparing herself for her travels to her family roots in South America, and later, Spain. I felt this spelt disaster for my toes and for those of my partner.

"'You see that is what we should do. It's active, we will meet people, and afterwards we can dance and have a drink. All for a fiver a time!' Complacently she leant back in her chair. Sarah had made up her mind and so we embarked on this with all the gusto of real dancing enthusiasts. We arrived at the entrance of the North London Polytechnic Hall and peered through the door, to be greeted by a barrage of 'Hello, hello... come in, come... your names, yes... Yes... that way.' We followed the officious young man down the corridor at a trot. When the music started we nearly jumped out of our skins. The gaggle of dancers began to jiggle from one foot to the other. Sarah and I were motionless. Sarah leant over to me, arms folded, and whispered, 'Who's the teacher...?'

"She needn't have asked. At that moment a swarthy, wrinkle-faced man and a bird-like woman flounced into the room. Clap clap. Sarah and I just looked at each other. We were obviously going to dance together. Above the music the instructors screeched the command 'Cooooooopyyyyyy!'

"I am not sure who led who, but with a swirl here and a stamp there we began. Trying at every turn to cover up compulsive giggles, we tracked the teaching couple like a cat chasing a mouse. Sarah and I clutched each other as we spun round, hoping through the blur that we weren't going to end up in a heap on the floor. Our toes began to throb, and, exhausted after an hour, we slumped on to some chairs.

"'Well, not quite what I expected', said Sarah trying to catch her breath. 'Where was all that sensuous stuff they mentioned in the advert? And the people – I know you already! All I've seen is a couple of gay men, two or three couples trying to get the spark back into their relationship, and three hopeful all-girl dancing partnerships like us. Where's the sensitive, caring-looking Latin type gone from the poster? He wasn't in the class. Fancy a drink?'

"Needless to say, we never returned to the Salsa class!"

FROM A POXY ROOM IN LONDON
Sarah writes home, 5th July 1988:
"Dearly beloved...

"I thought I would write, partly because I haven't done so for ages and partly because I thought you might like to have something interesting on the door mat when you got home. Only assuming you can get in the door after all those huge meals you've been having this last week. And don't go trying to tell me you worked it off on the mountainside, 'cos it won't wash.

"Talking of watery subjects, the weather has been crazy down here. By 4 o'clock it was thundering again. Beaumont is beautiful when the sun is out. Today they were mowing the lawns so that the smell was overpowering in a wet grassy kind of way. Today I sat by the fountain and watched the goldfish and it was really pleasant. Such a pity we have to come back to this dump of an evening.

"The course is very good though one of our tutors is annoying because she doesn't seem to know much about the subject beyond the notes. She often loses the attention of the class. Luckily the other tutor is much more with it and can take the jokes thrown at her much better.

"Sitting on my left I have a graduate from Hong Kong. He has perfect English and offered to book us for a Chinese meal in

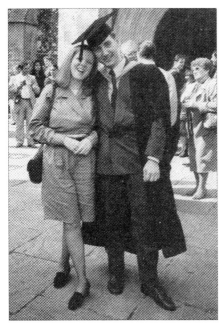

Sarah at Mark's graduation, 1991

Hounslow. We all made a fuss of him because he spoke to the restaurant in Cantonese, which will ensure we get well treated. Should be fun!

"At work I am joining a marketing/account department based at, wait for it, Feltham.

"The dance on Saturday was great fun and I was amazed at my stamina. I felt really special in my dress and I'm rather annoyed that we might not have any full length photos of me or Harriet dressed up. My frock was basically dark navy, boned bodice, full skirts with layered and ruffled blue net petticoats, off shoulder with straps going out across arms. Across bosom and straps large bows in navy lined inside with pale pink. Pale pink edge to outer petticoat. Ballerina length at front, full at back. Swirly and draping on stairs. What more could a girl want??

"The setting was all quite grand and it took me a couple of glasses of Bucks Fizz to stop feeling inadequate. We got the train to Market Harborough and played 'spot the co-party goer'. They were mostly boys in stripey shirts and Barbours. Taxis were laid on to the house which was in a terribly twee village called Melbourne. All like something out of Miss Marple or 'The Archers'. We changed in the village hall which doubles as a primary school.

"The loos were very low and marked 'Girls' and 'Boys'. The house had a driveway ankle deep in gravel. Built of stone with a scrumptious panelled staircase, stone window casements and window seats! I never did work out which one was Mr Alliance and Leicester, but the two bouncy castles were obviously his idea

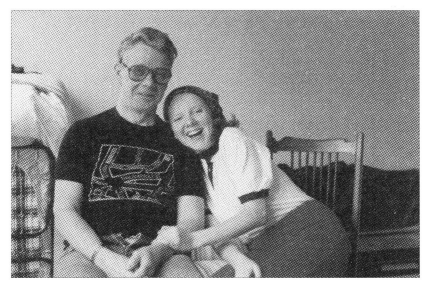

Bruce helped Sarah to decorate her 'poxy' flat!

as they were sponsored by his Building Society.

"Dinner was in a massive marquee in the garden, there were two hundred of us, cold buffet, then a jazz band and a disco. Round about 2am we started to get bored. The dashing men of our dreams hadn't turned up to chat although we had two of the nicest dresses in the place!

"Then breakfast at 4 30am. When we went to change, the hall was littered with bodies. The drive home was great but I had a scare when I noticed that our driver, Jo, was beginning to drop off! So I talked to her non-stop from then on. She hadn't drunk at all, but no sleep...

"One last piece of news. I now have a Filofax – aaah! We were given them on this course. I feel intimidated just looking at the darn thing.

"I must stop jabbering or you'll never get this till yonks after you get home.

"Lots of love, Sarah x x x"

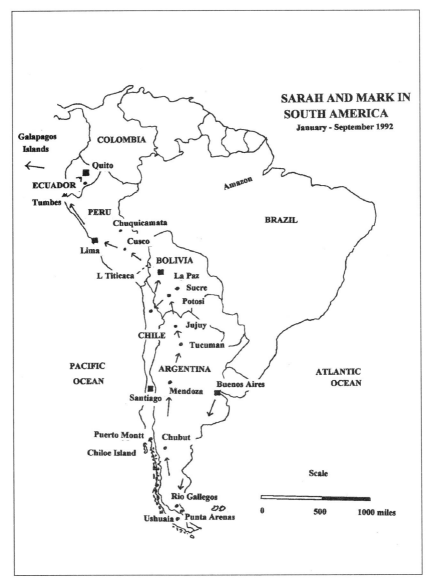

Arrowed route shows Sarah and Mark's journey

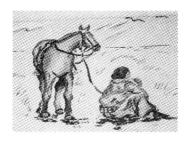

Chapter 6
THE GRAND TOUR
SOUTH AMERICA
1992

I travel for travel's sake. The great affair is to move.

Robert Louis Stevenson, Travels with a Donkey, 1879

ON 22 January 1992 Sarah and her brother Mark flew from London's Heathrow Airport to Buenos Aires. They would remain in South America until 25 September and would visit six different countries.

They had unexpected, as well as planned experiences. They saw wild life sanctuaries, glaciers and volcanoes. They reached Ushuaia, the world's most southerly city, and camped in the Tierro del Fuego National Park. They relaxed in thermal baths in Chile, and were confronted by armed guards with bullet proof vests and a list of 'of everyone that passeth'. There were cascades, geysers, ravines, a hill of seven colours, a silver mine, a drive across a salt lake, a hairy trip by boat, and a famously long train journey.

They were robbed and tear-gassed, were in Ecuador for the Presidential elections, and visited the Galapagos Islands and the Amazonian jungle.

Here is the outline itinerary of the trip made by Mark and Sarah, followed by some extracts from their correspondence to friends and family at home.

1992
ARGENTINA
Jan 22 Left Heathrow Airport for Buenos Aires
Feb 19 Left Buenos Aires
Feb 20 Arrived Chubut, Patagonia
Feb 21 Peninsula Valdes wild life sanctuary
Feb 25 Perito Moreno National Park
CHILE
Mar 3 Torres del Paine National Park
Mar 8 Milodon Cave
ARGENTINA
Mar 9 Rio Gallegos to Ushuaia
Mar 12 Camped in Tierra del Fuego National Park
CHILE
Mar 16 Puerto Natales – Punta Arenas
Mar 19 Ferry to Puerto Montt (4 days, 3 nights) visiting various islands
Mar 27 Ensenada, armed guards, volcano
Apr 8 Santiago
ARGENTINA
Apr 11 Mendoza
Apr 17 Through ravines to Molinos
Apr 19 Purnamarca, hill of seven colours
Apr 20 Across salt lake to Abra Pampa
Apr 23 Jujuy. Good Friday procession
BOLIVIA
May 1 Tarabuco market
May 2 -5 Potosi silver mine
May 7 Famous train journey,
28 hours instead of 14
CHILE
May 8-11 Calama, valley of the geysers and Valley of the Moon
May 18 Chuquicamata copper mine, 660m, deepest hole in the world
May 20 Rock designs, including the Giant of Atacama
May 23-25 Lauca National Park, ice, flamingoes and vizcachas
BOLIVIA
May 27 La Paz, collect mail
Jun 6 Bag gone missing
Jun 7 Copacabana, Isla del Sol
PERU
Jun 18 Corpus Christi festival at Cusco
Jun 21 Raqchi dance festival
Jun 25 Lima

ECUADOR
Jun 26 Tear-gassed at Tumbes
Jun 5-9 Quito, Presidential elections
Jun 15-27 Galapagos Islands
Aug 2-6 Amazon jungle
COSTA RICA
Aug 29- Sept 25
25 Sept 08.50 Sarah arrives at Heathrow airport London

EXPLORING SOUTH AMERICA
Edited correspondence and diary extracts from Mark and Sarah

Postcard from Sarah, Chubut, Argentina, 23 February 1992:
"We have spent a lovely three days seeing the Welsh towns and seeing the sea-lions, sea-elephants and penguins. We really blew our first week's budget, but it was so exciting. The male sea elephants are like great grey slugs, only moving when the tide caught up with them. The sea lions we saw from a boat, all having their siestas at the water's edge, and the penguins we would actually walk among. Mark adds 'Weather's here, wish you were fine,' well, something like that! It's lovely down here, so much to see and so little time to see it. Lots of luv."

Letter from Mark, Calafate Youth Hostel, Southern Argentina, 25 February 1992:
"This country is so large and diverse, it's so unbelievable. Our journey south from Buenos Aires started really well. The bus was 40 minutes late and we had to wait in a steaming heat of 41°C. I don't know how my climatic system is going to cope.

"Once we left Buenos Aires the countryside was flat all the way. It's not as boring as its sounds. In the distance we could see an amazing thunderstorm lighting up all the clouds. It rained on and off for the whole journey of 15 hours. We arrived at Puerto Madryn in torrential rain and it didn't stop all night. We booked in at our hotel, small, quiet, 'cleanish' and hot water (the vital point). We then went out armed with all our waterproof gear and walking boots. It pissed it down. After half an hour all the streets were flooded, we were soaked, and would you believe it, enjoying ourselves. I've never seen rain like it. Around 250mm fell during 24 hrs which is a hell of a lot when you put it all in a town near the sea, at the bottom of a hill! We seemed to spend half the night trying to cross roads, at one point we even got a lift from a car to the other side of the road.

"The next day we went on our first trip, to the national park on the Peninsula Valdes. It was amazing, the road there was mostly dirt track, and when we eventually reached the peninsula we saw an amazing sea lion colony sunbathing on the beach. They were so lovely, especially with all their babies, messing about and playing all the time.

"We saw penguins at Punto Tombo, further down the coast. It was incredible. We arrived at this place in the middle of nowhere, after getting a puncture and breaking down on the way, and when the bus drove to the car park we were surrounded by penguins. Apparently there are around ½ million penguins here at the height of the breeding season and I could well believe it. The path you walked on weaved in and out of all the bushes under which the penguins nested and you had to be very careful in case you trod on one. They were so funny, especially all the babies who were beginning to lose all their fluffy feathers. The noise they made was really weird, they brayed like donkeys.

"We got a bus to Rio Gallegos. You would just love this place. I have been sitting beside a lagoon which is on the shore of Lago Argentino, the largest lake in Argentina, the third largest in the world. It is surrounded on three sides by glorious mountains with the town of Calafate behind me. I have taken a photo from where I am sat so you can see the view I am experiencing.

"Calafate is a small town of about 3,000 people, in the middle of nowhere. The next town is four hours away. We took a trip to the Moreno Glacier, which is one of the few advancing in the world. It was so exciting watching the glacier, like having a geography lesson come true.

"The glacier in total covers an area of some $150km_2$ on one side. It comes down from the mountain and plunges into the start of Lago Argentina, which is a beautiful milky blue colour. We sat near the face, and watched as large chunks of the face fell into the water. Considering the face is 60m high, they created quite a wave. It was so difficult to tear ourselves away as the glacier kept emitting incredible sounds as it cracked internally."

Letter from Mark, Torres del Paine, Chile:
"We have not been in a town big enough or at the right time of day to find a post office. This is being written in a *refugio*, one of the campers' huts dotted all round the national parks.

"This one is slightly more upmarket. It has a toilet, a range on which to cook, and even beds! Well, you could call

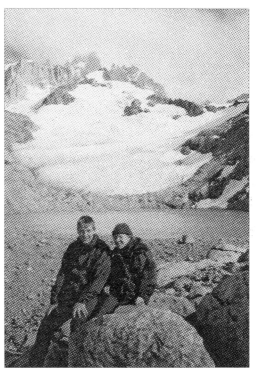

Torres del Paine, Chile

them beds. They consist of a sort of sloping roof, as wide as you are long, so you sleep at an angle (hopefully sleep anyway!), that's if you can avoid all the nails in the planks. I look like a seasoned traveller, haven't had a shower for five days, not even a wash, my hair is all standing on end, I've got a tan (not by sun but by wind), and the beard is coming along well!

"The standard of living in Chile is a lot higher than that of Argentina. the main difference being the cars, there were lots of nice American jeeps, Chevrolets, and even the odd BMW, with a sprinkling of Beetles to top it off. Judging by the amount of unpaved roads down here I don't think they ever heard of tarmac. The nearest town to here is four hours away."

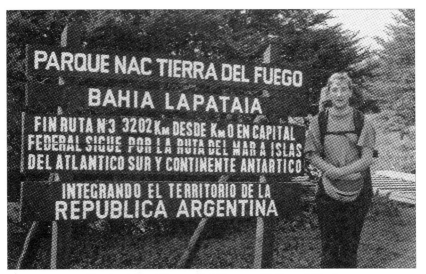

Mark at the Tierra del Fuego National Park

Letter from Sarah, Hotel Colonial, Rio Gallegos, Argentina:

"We spent a night camping in the Tierro del Fuego National Park. At dusk we were beaver watching. We sat by a large dam hoping to see them there, where the two lodges were. Instead Mark spotted the first one downstream, beyond the dam. We crept up but he never saw us, although he would circle round, looking directly at us and sniffing. Then we saw him again with two others. Two of them came to shore to drink and munch on greenery and Mark got to within a metre of one of them. I wandered up to the dam and saw one pull himself out of the water, clamber laboriously up and over the dam and into the water again. He took one of the freshly cut leafy branches floating in the pond in his mouth and swam with it to store it.

"Mark makes me laugh a lot and organises us re the cooking stoves and things. I try hard not to be a feeble female but he takes over, so fine! And all the fires he's been able to light! 7th heaven!"

Letter from Mark, Punta Arenas, Chile, 26 March 92:

"We visited the Salesian Museum, set up by priests who originally came to protect the local Indians from being wiped out by the settlers. It was like walking though somebody's private collection of junk. Boxes of soil (?) and stuffed animals littered the place, which smelled of moth balls, scattered all over the exhibition. There was even a doddery old priest wandering around with a stuffed penguin! That night is started snowing, and heavily. Summer in Punta Arenas!

"We took a boat to Quinchas Island, off the eastern side of Chiloe Island, Chile. Our sailing was at 5.55 am. It was cold and windy – a perfect day for sailing! The boat was full of backpackers all doing the same thing. Being primarily a cargo boat, the deck was full of lorries carrying sheep and cows, all packed in like sardines, unable to move. What a horrible way to travel. Even worse than that was our cabin, which slept 12, and was a portacabin fixed to the deck and was right behind the cows. So our lovely fresh sea air in the morning smelled like we had been staying on a farm. We only hit the sea and its swell at one point.

"There weren't too many casualties. Sarah and I escaped with the aid of some seasickness pills.

"The scenery we passed through was lovely, with so many islands covered with thick green forests. At one point three dolphins came up to the boat and swam in the bow wave. Even saw more penguins and some albatross as well."

Letter from Mark, Ensenada, Chilean lake district:

"We are on a campsite close to Lake Llanquihue. The skies are clear and blue and we have an amazing view of the snow capped Volcan Osorno, an extinct volcano.

(LATER)... just watching the last rays of sunlight hit the volcano!..."

Letter from Sarah, in a 'Refugio', Volcan Osorno, Chile:

"We are in grand isolation, more or less, half way up a dormant volcano. We are not in our tent but in a rather lovely alpine type cottage used by walkers and climbers in the summer and by skiers in the winter. We are about 11km from the nearest anywhere, which isn't anywhere much as it doesn't even have a proper shop. It does, of course, have its *carabinieri* post – 'and the Lord sayeth unto Chile and Argentina, wherever two or three huts are gathered together in my name, let there be soldiers with bullet-proof vests, sub-machine guns, and a list of everyone that passeth'. At least here they do seem to have a purpose, as they seem to double up as the mountain rescue service. About five years ago six climbers were stranded up here, when the guards came in a helicopter to try and find them they crashed the 'copter into the mountain in the cloud. The six climbers froze to death overnight. They were like this, the guy here told me, tapping the iron of the range in the kitchen, 'congelated'.

"The hedges here are groaning with blackberries so both of us have stained hands from picking them. I spotted a farmhouse on the way up selling honey. There is a hotel in the village which has wonderful German apple cake, so we have plenty of treats in store. We managed to camp on the beach of the huge Lago Llanquihue and had a front of stalls view of a magnificent sunset which coloured the glaciers on the cone of the volcano delicate pinks, thrusting the crevasses into dark shadow."

Letter from Mark, near Osorno, Chilean lake district, 5 April 1992:

"At Peulla we camped in the garden of the *guardaparque*. He seemed too friendly if anything and his son followed us around for most of the day. Nice at first, but got annoying very quickly. As Sarah said, there's only so much small chat you can have with a kid who is seven. What is the Spanish for 'How do you fancy a trip to the bottom of the lake with a pair of lead boots?'"

Letter from Sarah, Jujuy, Chile, 23 April 1992:

"We had breakfast on a salt lake and drove on to it to see where men were scraping salt. We stayed in a little *hospedaje* wedged in under a mountain, which was coloured orange, purple, pink and green, a really weird sight to wake up to as we had arrived in the dark. We have seen herds of llama and *vicuña* and Indian ladies in red and green shawls, hats, layered skirts and baby on back. We saw a Good Friday procession of the cross and we've seen the ruins of an enormous pre-Incaic village where I almost put my hand on a snake."

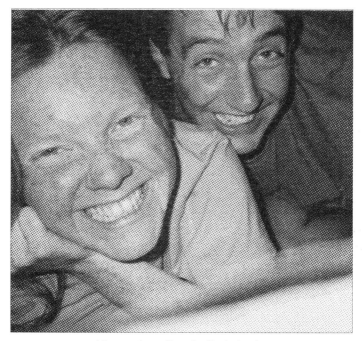

Happy together in their tent...

Letter from Mark, Sucre, Bolivia, 25 April 1992:

"Here we are in a new country. Bolivia is the poorest country in South America, yet the people here are some of the most colourful and friendly that we have met so far. It is also by far one of the cheapest.

"We left for Mendoza in Argentina on 11 April. The drive over the Andes was just amazing. We were blessed with glorious blue skies and incredible views for the whole journey. We began the big climb up from the Rio Colorado, and we could see the road zigzagging up the mountain. On the map the road here is just one great big blur because of all the hairpin bends to climb up. It was on this journey that we saw our first cacti, some of them were even flowering! The colours in the mountains changed all the time, from deep reds, to greens, browns and greys. You just didn't want to leave!

"Fed up with buses, and not knowing how they will run over

the Easter weekend, we have hired a car, a little Fiat called Cecil. We set off for Cafayate on Thursday. Such a lovely journey, along a valley like a rain forest, coming out into a very dry and barren landscape. It was all very beautiful, with such wonderful colours in all the rocks. We stopped at Quilmes, the most southerly Inca ruins ever found in Argentina. The site was on the side of a barren valley and about 1½ kms long. It's hard to believe that this valley could support such a large town. The whole area is like one big desert, with cacti growing in forests, hundreds of them!

"We headed for Abra Pampa, passing our highest point yet at 4170 metres. We crossed the Tropic of Capricorn, our first time ever."

Postcard from Mark and Sarah, Sucre, Bolivia, 28 April 1992:
"We've been having fun though Mark was icky poo yesterday. Could it be to do with the nine bottles of beer he sunk with another English guy? No, it was the dodgy Chinese food we ate. Anyway, better now."

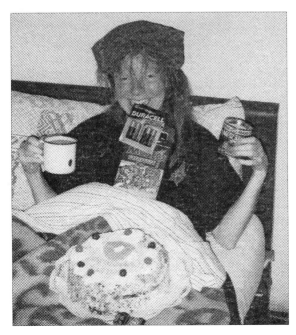

Sarah's birthday on May 10, 1992: Mark's nickname for her was "Duracell" (because of the copper hair), so he bought her a packet together with a pre-ordered birthday cake and some expensive coffee. Another present was the red scarf on her head.

Postcard from Mark and Sarah, Valle de la Luna, Chile, 13 May 1992:
"I'm always kind to Mark when I start a card and leave him a small space in which to repeat what I have just said in a different way. How come he always leaves me half the card? Sarah"

Postcard from Sarah, Iquique, Chile, 19 May 1992:
"Gloriously hot in the day and not too bitter at night as it is only 2400m. We visited incredible geysers, bathed in Garden of Eden like thermal springs, camped at full moon in a desert valley of weird wind-carved rocks and sand dunes, walked to pre-Incaic ruins on mountain tops and admired sunset over a string of volcanoes."

Letter from Sarah, La Paz, Bolivia, 27 May 1992:
"It is Mother's Day today, so everyone is wandering around clutching single red roses, gunky cakes and execrable posters and ceramic things.

"It's a strange existence, meeting people then moving on. Most people you are really glad to leave behind, a few you feel you would actually like to keep in touch with, and one or two you really regret having to leave. One evening we stayed up late with three other guys arguing politics – a Norwegian traveller we also met, he and I stayed up half the night talking with an Argentine chap we met on our tour of the mine at Potosi.

"We left at 4am to see the geysers at dawn when the ground is still frozen and the bubbling hot water gives off steam that goes rainbow colours as the sun shines through it. We boiled eggs in one geyser pool.

"We went to the Lauca National Park. -10 deg C at night in the tent – wearing all your clothes and ice on the inside of the tent. But we camped on the lake with flamingoes and dozens of other birds and *vizcacha*, which are like a sort of rabbit cum wallaby. They like to sun themselves on the rocks. From there we hitched on a lorry the 12 or so hours to the main La Paz highway. An amazing bone-juddering journey on the WORST road across the Altiplano. You have never seen two such dusty individuals."

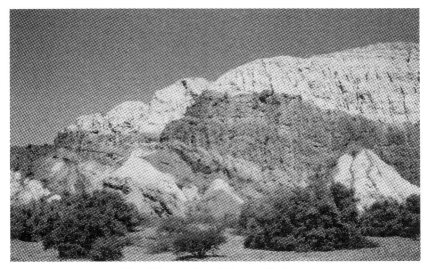

The 'Mountain of Seven Colours'

Letter from Mark, Copacabana, Bolivia, 7 June 1992:

"Thank God we have finally left La Paz. By the time this letter reaches you we will probably be in Quito soaking up the sun. Jealous?

"It's weird, but as every day goes by, we keep thinking of things that we need that were stolen in La Paz. Like a calculator, penknife, scissors, sun tan lotion, and me tuthbrush! and my DIARY. If the people who nick bags from the street knew of the heartache that they cause, I wonder if they would still do it? Probably yes; it is a bloody easy way to make lots of money.

"We have been to Lago Chungara, the highest lake of its size in the world, at 4500m bloody high, bloody windy and bloody cold. The whole area is spectacular. The shore's edge was covered with birds, with some pink flamingoes thrown in for good measure. On one side of the lake opposite our camp site there was a snow-capped volcano called Parinacota, with a second one behind it. To the right were more mountains, not covered in snow as all the others were, but with the most beautiful colours, browns, reds, oranges, just like those bottles you get at the seaside which are full of multi-coloured sands. At sunset they were just out of this world. We went for a walk along the lake just before it got dark, and the place was full of *vizcacha*, those little animals. sitting on rocks, like rabbits but with long bushy tails. They hopped about like little kangaroos!

"Once the sun goes down it doesn't half get cold. We went to bed in the tent at around 8 o'clock, fully clothed in about three layers, and we were still cold. We woke up in the morning with ice on the inside of the tent from our breath, all our water frozen and the pots which had been left to soak overnight like solid blocks of ice. Here April, May and June are the coldest months and the temperature can fall to around -25°C, luckily the lowest we had was -10°C, definitely cold enough for us. The National Park ranger showed us a picture of when they caught a condor. This bird kills the alpaca and the *vicuña*, and this one they got had a wing span of 3m, pretty big, eh. Princess Anne even came to the park in 1991, and the ranger showed us his visitor book with her signing herself as 'Anne' and occupation as 'HRH'. Funny to think of an HRH going to the same places we have, especially when they are in the middle of nowhere.

"La Paz, the capital of Bolivia, is a beautiful city in the weirdest of settings. When you approach it the only sign that you are getting nearer is the sight of the incredible mountain Illimani and the poorer areas. Then all of a sudden the plain ends and there is this amazing canyon with skyscrapers filling the bottom and houses built all the way around, climbing up the steep sides. A gorgeous site, and lovely to see a whole city in one breathtaking view!

"La Paz has a mixture of cultures. Walking down the same street you will have the businessmen/women in their suits, and the *campesinos* (country people) with the women wearing their bowler hats and multi-layered skirts. They make up 70% of the population of Bolivia and most of them speak in the own dialect, whether it be Aymara or Quechua as well as Spanish, and most of them speak all three! Puts a person to shame. La Paz is full of wonderful markets, people selling goods by the road. You don't need supermarkets here, you can get everything you need, from a toothbrush to a light bulb, on the side of the road.

"We visited a set of ancient ruins at Tiwanaku, from the now extinct Tiwanaku tribe which dominated the whole area for 1000s of years before the Incas showed up. It was a gorgeous place, now preserved as a national monument. Some of the walls were over 5m high. There are large slabs of rock used as altars, which weigh hundreds of tons. No one knows how they ever got the rocks to the site. It is even more of a mystery considering the Tiwanaku didn't have the wheel!

"The highlight of the day had to be the vicious llama. A big white cuddly thing with long eyelashes which had a rope attached to it, presumably so it could be tethered up. As we walked by it along the path all of a sudden it came running up to us and jumped on Sarah's back. I reckon it was trying to mount her, but that is only my opinion! Needless to say we ran off, only later on in the day, whilst we were looking at other ruins, it came running round a hill, aiming straight for us. Sarah screamed. I threw stones and it stopped. We thought it was a personal vendetta, but it proved us wrong by attacking everyone within a 1km radius. Everyone we talk to who has visited Tiwanaku has had the same experience with 'the vicious llama.'"

Letter from Mark, Quito, Ecuador, 1 July 1992:

"Our first couple of days in Cusco were spent finding out where all the best shops were. We made our best discovery yet, a pub called 'Cross Keys' run by an Englishman from Manchester and his Peruvian wife. An excellent place with a really good atmosphere, and what was more important, a Happy Hour (even had a dart board as well, but couldn't get on it for the foreigners)! We seemed to spend the beginning of nearly every evening there.

"Not that I drank of course, I didn't want to let my halo slip, but don't ask Sarah because she will only lie and tell you different – who am I trying to kid, eh!

"We headed off for the big adventure of our stay in Peru, a visit to Machu Picchu. We caught the local train. The tourist one cost over $70 when the local one cost £8. The countryside we passed through was basically jungle with thick forests climbing up the sides of the mountains which surrounded the track. Just beautiful! On the way we went to the weird little town of Agua Caliente, with its one and only high street consisting of the railway line, with most of the restaurants and shops fronting on to it. We found a hotel called Gringo Bill's. The room we eventually got can only be described as 'different', and worth the extra that we paid. Everything in the room was purple, the walls, curtains, bed spread, and even the number above the door. We had windows on three sides and a balcony on two, overlooking the town. And to top it all off, a very 'hippie' type erotic painting at the foot of the beds, taking up most of the wall. Not the sort of room you share with your sister!

"The next morning we set off early for Machu Picchu, aiming to get there before most of the tourists arrived on the train. We walked the 2km or so down the line to the Machu Picchu station, where a road and a footpath climb up the side of the mountain.

We had missed the first bus so we ended up walking, or more precisely climbing, the 500m straight up to the ruins. As we climbed up we had glimpsed terracing and the edges of the ruins most of the time, but when we eventually passed through the entrance gate and saw the ruins in their entirety, it just took your breath away. At last we got to see in real life the sight that before we had only ever seen in books and magazines. There is only one word to describe it, and that is BEAUTIFUL.

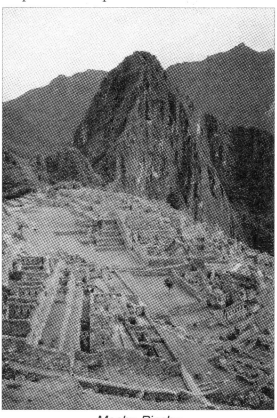

Machu Picchu

67

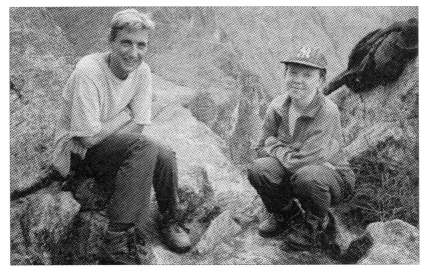

Sitting on top of Huayna Picchu

"We really didn't want to leave Machu Picchu, a magical place. But as it started to rain that sort of made up our minds for us. We began the long climb down. We rewarded ourselves when we reached the town by going to the thermal baths, after which the town is named. It was really nice lying there in the steaming water, watching the sun set and seeing the stars rise. A perfect end to a perfect day!

"The next day we went to Alantaytambo. It had another spectacular set of ruins, with the main section consisting of baths. An intricate series of underground channels, and some even cut into solid rock, culminating in beautiful shallow baths. Some even had water still running through them, still falling precisely down the hole carved in the floor. We wanted to be back in Cusco before dark. We knew that it was Corpus Christi when we got back, but I don't think any of us were prepared for the amount of people who filled the town. You could hardly walk down any of the main streets for food stalls and people, and the main plaza was impossible to get through. We got to the hotel, dumped all our gear, and braved the crowds.

"We spent the rest of the evening working our way through the streets eating and drinking, but not being quite brave enough to try the roast guinea-pig. The worst thing is that it looked like a guinea pig including sticky out teeth and claws, which some people used as toothpicks – Yuck!

"In the main plaza in Cusco there was a Light and Sound show, part of the festival week. A couple of million people crammed tightly in a small space. The first time either of us have felt so vulnerable in such a situation. You were just so powerless against a heaving mass of people. It culminated in a spectacular firework display, the largest Cusco had ever seen, and there were plenty of oohs and aahs from the crowd. That was followed by more crushing as everyone tried to leave at the same time!

"After being crushed in so many crowds, we didn't really want to see another procession. But the one in the Plaza de Armas was so well organised and involved so many people that we decided to see the main ceremony at Sacsayhuaman (pronounced like Sexy-woman), the old Inca fortress which overlooks Cusco. We found a good spot on the fortress walls (which was made out of huge rocks, some weighing over 300 tons each), and sat down waiting for 'the show'. It was just spectacular, with hundreds of people co-ordinated into a fascinating display, acting out the history of the Incas. The show lasted two hours, with the winners from Raquichi finishing off the day with their show. We left at that point, having seen enough dancing and wailing to last us a lifetime!

"We went on by plane to Lima, a place that nobody was looking forward to, what with bombs, curfews and pickpockets. The whole city was full of army, all armed to the teeth. A little bit unnerving to say the least! In Peru nearly every other car you see is a Beetle, most of the taxis being one. Even had a ride in one!

"We got a taxi to Agua Verde, a town on the border of Ecuador with Peru. You couldn't tell where you had left Peru and entered Ecuador because the town just kept on going, with street stalls everywhere. We relaxed in a nice restaurant, and both started falling asleep until something woke us up! Two men came running down the street, chased by a crowd throwing stones and bottles. They ran into the police station and the guards locked the gate. Nothing much happened for a while so I went to the loo, only to be interrupted by shouts and screams. I rushed out, only to breathe in a great big cloud of tear-gas, which virtually blinded me in a couple of seconds. Everyone, including Sarah, was out the back dousing themselves in water. Our first day in Ecuador, and we get tear-gassed! That definitely woke us up for the rest of the afternoon, the best thing was that the police didn't have gas masks, so when they let off the canisters they were affected as well! Good move!

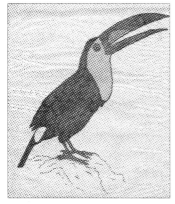

Sarah loved observing and drawing birds – it seems appropriate to include her drawing of a S American bird, the Sulphur-breasted Toucan

"After arriving in Quito, the capital of Ecuador, we were taken out for a gorgeous lunch. A Hawaiian place where all the waiters wore white gloves (nothing else?) when they served you, and all the *agua mineral con gas* was free. They just came round topping your glass up.

"After stuffing ourselves we drove for about half an hour to the north of Quito to the point at which the Equator crosses. An incredible place with this massive monument, topped off with a globe on its side so that the Equator ran down the monument, with a line on the ground passing through a small precinct. Amazing, standing astride the line, with one half of you in the northern hemisphere and the other half in the south. The big question is, does the water in a basin directly over the Equator go down the plughole straight?

"We have confirmed our trips to the Galapagos Islands and the Amazon. We have an eight-day tour of the islands, followed by a boat trip in a canoe in the jungle for five days, and from there up to Costa Rica. And then home!"

The following letter 'to Mummy and Daddy, from Sarah' (dated 20 July 1992) was sent from the yacht *Española* during Sarah's and Mark's eight-day tour of the Galapagos Islands off Ecuador:

"My mind is being addled by too much idling on a boat and far too much good eating. Our cook works minor miracles in the tiny galley. We are having a wonderful time. Thank you so much Mummy for making sure we came here. We are on a small but neat boat with a crew of three; Captain, cook, sailor, plus a guide and six other passengers, Swedish, British and Swiss. Our guide is excellent with good English save the odd hilarious Spanglishism, eg 'the sea is very moved' ('*movido*' = rough). Today we swam in a pool, partly cut off from the sea by a lava bridge, with fur seals. We were too many for them to cope with so they bustled off, but we later watched one having superb fun in a sink hole where the water rose and fell several metres with each wave. We could get anxious as he didn't surface for two or three waves, and then there would be the flap of a tail and down he would go again. Tomorrow we should see penguins – on the Equator – seems crazy, no?"

Letter from Sarah to Mummy and Daddy, Los Rios, Quito, Ecuador, 14 August 1992:
I am loathe to head off to Costa Rica and being with lots of people again. I am loving having my own room, pottering, doing my (Spanish) lessons, writing my diary, reading (crisis looming as I've finished my book and need to do a swap). I have given myself a long overdue image overhaul, bought myself a T-shirt and trousers, and had 6cms lopped off my hair. And it's still a few cms below my shoulders!

The owner of the *cabañas* (cabins) where we stayed in the jungle invited me to his eldest son's wedding reception on the 22nd, which is another reason why I'm in two minds about leaving that afternoon for Costa Rica. The problem is that the invitation was issued late at night after a few Cuba *libres* and I'm somewhat reliant on meeting our guide, Julio, before the event, in order to know the hows and wherefores of going. And he seems to have disappeared off t'ut jungle again unexpectedly. Bloody latins. Still I incline to forgive him as he is very good looking and dances very well.

Lots of love, *besos y abrazos*. Sarah
THAT'S IT FOLKS!

Mark's diary for the Trip – from Quito, Ecuador to the Galapagos, 13 July 1992:

"**Day One:** Well at last the moment we've both been waiting for – our trip to the Galapagos Islands and as I sit here writing, the whole world around us is moving – the bell in the galley is swinging from side to side and stars keep appearing and then disappearing from view.

"We caught the plane from Quito to Baltra on the Islands and when we boarded the ship there was an incredible lunch waiting for us, and the food standard proved to be that high for the next few days. The weather proved not particularly warm but our guide informed us that we had arrived in the changeover period from the dry to the wet season, though apparently this is good for the animals.

"Our first destination was a beach on Santa Cruz (Holy Cross) Island, the main one. A gorgeous beach with white sand, with pelicans flying around everywhere. Frigate birds looking remarkably like pterodactyls in flight and even sea lions swimming around just off the beach. We also saw our first marine iguana, the first of many. Had a really relaxing time, went for a bit of snorkelling, it was just like swimming around in a tropical fish tank, with shoals of small shiny fish parting as you swam between them. When we went back to the boat we even had tea and biscuits waiting for us – very civilised, I must admit!

"**Day Two:** Early the next morning we set off for Plarzas, a couple of islands just off the eastern side of Santa Cruz, where there are a couple of colonies of sea lions. The tender took us to the small jetty that had been built and as we got nearer the steps began to move and baby seals jumped into the water to greet us. It was just incredible as we landed, you could get so close to the animals – within a couple of feet of some of them. They were just so beautiful (and smelly). They were so docile and seem to accept human beings, with the young pups even being a little curious. The place was just crawling with wildlife, we saw numerous land iguanas, marine iguanas, Lewa lizards, hundreds of Sally Lightfoot crabs, blue-footed boobies – all incredible and beautiful in their own little way – just seeing this lot was worth the trip.

"We then headed across the open sea and our first very rough

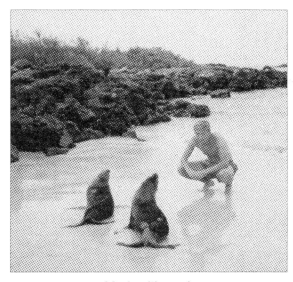

Mark with seals

water to Santa Fe Island which has its own little natural harbour, with clear blue water. It had a lovely sandy beach occupied by another sea lion colony. We just spent time sitting there watching them and after a short walk came back to this spot to have a swim, and we were even joined by a couple of baby sea lions – like a dream come true. On the journey back to the Espanola we saw the outline of a sting ray.

"**Day Three:** We had a six-hour journey to Floreana to see the colony of Pink Flamingos, the largest on the islands. We were told that when young the birds are a white colour, turning pink as they grow older and eat their main food, small shrimp. The other side of the island there was a beach which was pure white in colour, formed by the fish over the years eating the white coral. After another lovely lunch we went to Post Barrel Bay. We went on a short trip in the launch around the coast avoiding all the rocks, to a small beach. Just behind which is this incredible collection of bits and pieces around a couple of old wooden barrels *(see picture on page 77)*. What people do is put post cards in one of them and as people arrive, you look through the pile and see if there are any in your country. The idea is you are supposed to post them when you get back home. We then snorkelled in a place called the Devil's Crown, an outcrop of rock just off the coast, looking remarkably like a crown. The sea was really too choppy and even though it was sheltered, the current too strong to really enjoy the swim.

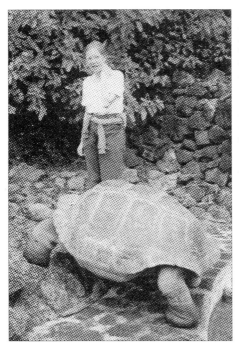
Sarah and tortoise

"**Day Four:** We went back to the boat and set off for Puerto Ayora on the southern end of Santa Cruz where the next morning we visited the Charles Darwin station, set up about 50 years ago in order to protect the Giant Tortoises which were being gradually wiped out because of human intervention. There was an excellent information centre which explained the origins of the islands and of the animals which now inhabit them. We then headed off for the areas where they keep the tortoises. Nowadays they collect most of the eggs from around the islands and keep the animals for a couple of years until their shells are hard enough to resist attacks, so they can fend for themselves.

"Then we went for the most incredible sight ever, the Giant Tortoises. They are just so big, about a metre long and almost as high. They can actually walk quite fast, not bad for animals that they reckon are about 150 years old. Their fighting was also quite un-energetic, consisting of stretching their necks to see who could reach the highest, and the loser had to move out of the way. They were just so funny, creaking and groaning as they moved along. There is another tortoise of about the same age which is the only surviving animal of his species. He can't mate with the other breeds, so he is living out his time all on his own on an island, and his name, 'Lonely George'.

"In the afternoon we went to the centre of the island to see a wonderful geological formation consisting of two massive holes a couple of hundred metres wide and about a hundred metres deep formed during a volcanic eruption when a whole load of gas escaped making the top surface collapse. As we were walking through the trees we even saw an owl sitting in a bush preening itself. It is called a Short Eared Owl and is one of only two species of owls on the island and the only one that is out during the day.

"**Day Five:** an early crossing to Seymour Island, mainly a bird colony with Frigate and Blue Footed Boobies – plus the odd sea lion of course!). The birds, especially on Seymour, are totally fearless of humans, with the paths going very near to nesting sites. The male Frigates were showing off their beautiful red necks – we were so lucky to see them as we are nearing the end of the mating season. As well as displaying their pouches, when they sight a female they turn their heads upward, plus wings, and shake them vigorously. If the female is attracted and lands, the pair may wave their heads together and the male sometimes puts his wings around the female. After this we had a short spell whilst waiting for a new passenger, and caught up on sunbathing, getting pink as flamingos.

In the afternoon we headed for Tortuga Negra where we took the dingy into some mango groves, totally surrounded by water. It was like the films you see about the wetlands in America, taking the boat through small clearings and coming across another clearing. This was populated with sea turtles. At first we could only see the shadows in the water, but as we got further into the groves and the water became calmer, we could see them a lot more clearly. we drifted through the water without the engine on and they came a lot closer. Despite their size they were so graceful and quick in the water. Occasionally they would come to the surface and push their heads out and then slide back down into the water. There were massive sting rays, hugs shoals of Manta Rays and at one shallow point there were even five or six White Tipped Sharks, each a couple of metres long.

"**Day Six:** the area is more sheltered and the seas a lot calmer. On the island of Rabida there was another large flamingo colony, and the beach on this island a different glorious red colour, again with more sea lions and pelicans. We paddled in the water trying to attract the sea lions. Only one came anywhere near, a large female – definitely a bit frightening when they come at you at full pelt, only turning away right at the last minute. In the afternoon we went to San Salvador island, where there was a black volcanic beach. Owing to the effects of the El Niño current coming up from the Peruvian coast, the water temperatures have been lowered to 1°C, killing the plankton on which the marine iguana feed. This has had an unfortunate effect on the marine iguana colony, and we saw many dead animals over the beach and rocks. When we got back to the boat everyone was pleased as a large fish had been caught; not only this but later the captain and the sailor went off in the boat and returned a couple of hours later with dinner for the next couple of weeks: two fresh skinned goats, caught on the island (with their bare hands) to make our day complete, just before sunset a group of about four dolphins came swimming into the bay – just beautiful!

"**Day Seven:** Sullivan Bay: with its newest geological formations in the islands, a lava flow only 120 years old, the only place in the world outside of Hawaii that you can find this particular formation, rather like rope formations all over the surface – rather dangerous walking over it without shoes (Ah! Ah!). here we also saw the Galapagos penguins, the third smallest in the world and very very cute.

"**Day Eight:** our last day on the boat and a very early start, visiting Daphne Island, before breakfast and before sunrise. We scrambled up the side of the volcano weaving in and out of the Masked Boobies that nest on the island, so fascinating with their funny whistling calls and the weird way they walk. There were also many Frigate birds with their bright red pouches puffed out in full glory, visible even to us from our high vantage point.

"Puerto Ayara on the Islands: a lovely lazy day on Tortuga Bay, with the walk there seeming to take forever, walking through some pretty scenery with lava lizards littering the path, scattering whenever we came near. We began to hear the breakers crashing onto the beach and soon glimpsed the ocean. When we got to the beach the colour was incredible, a pure white along its whole

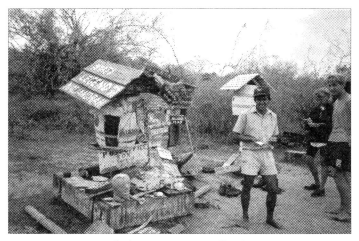

Galapagos post-office!

length, so bright that it almost blinded you as you walking along it. There were millions of crabs, all half out and half in their holes just about the water line.

"The following day we went on a horse ride with a group of people. Only one of us had ridden a horse before for any length of time. It was good fun watching the remainder of us trying to get aboard. The horses were all very docile and walked at a nice steady pace. The saddles left a little bit to be desired though, lumps of wood held on with bits of rope – very comfy! We rode to the tortoise reserve set deep into the forest, lovely, with moss hanging down from the trees, surrounded by fields of elephant grass, banana trees, avocado trees, papaya trees and much much more. We saw several Vermilion Fly Catchers with their bright red chests sitting in the bushes beside the path. After a lovely break we got back on the horses and after two hours of pain arrived back in Santa Rosa, feeling very much the worse for the wear, but having thoroughly enjoyed our adventure.. By the way, are all cowboys sterile? 'Cause it ain't half painful down below!"

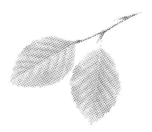

Chapter 7
VIGO, SPAIN
1993 – 1995

The sum of human wisdom is not contained in any one language, and no single language is capable of expressing all forms and degrees of human comprehension

Ezra Pound, The ABC of Reading, 1934

This section is written by Andrea Lyons:
The first contact I had with Sarah was with her laugh. I was sitting in the lounge of my new home at Vigo in northern Spain with a few other 'new' English language teachers, all trying to get to know each other and all no doubt feeling just as nervous and excited as myself.

The door intercom sounded and Frances, a teacher already living in the flat, went to welcome the last teacher to arrive and join our group. I knew there was a strong possibility that this person could turn out to be my flat mate as there was one room left and it seemed that other new teachers had already tentatively agreed to find accommodation together. As I was wondering what she would be like and whether or not we would be compatible as flat mates and maybe even good friends, the most amazing laugh started to echo down the long narrow corridor and fill the lounge where we were sitting. It wasn't a high pitched tinkle or a nervous giggle, but a proper, throaty, full blown 'chuck everything into it'

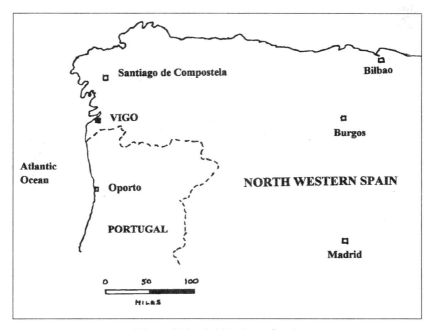

Map of North Western Spain

kind of laugh that immediately put me at ease and made me think there might be some fun times ahead. Then a flash of red appeared in the doorway and there was Sarah standing there with a beaming smile. I felt myself beaming back.

I often thank my lucky stars that Sarah decided to take that last room in the flat. It wasn't even a particularly nice room – quite cell-like, really, with a double bed and a large wardrobe that, between them, took up nearly all of the space. It had a large window that looked on to an inner courtyard of the block of flats and also looked directly across to a window in the flat opposite. It wasn't a courtyard that one immediately imagines where the sun peeps down and geraniums and ivy grow, but simply a hollow tube to allow extra air and light into the flats, where all the bathrooms backed on to, and where an odd sock and bits of litter lay at the bottom.

Sarah, to my amazement, did not seem bothered. She immediately took down the gaudy unattractive Spanish pictures and

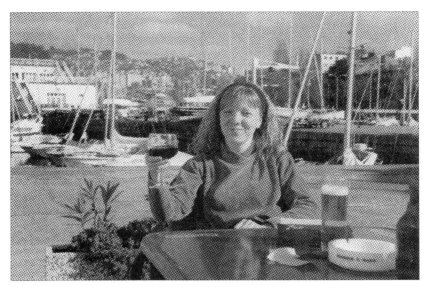

Sarah at the marina

ornaments hanging on the walls and started to replace them with photos of her family, and postcards from friends in other exotic parts of the world. I instantly came to realise that Sarah had come to Spain with the complete intention of throwing her whole self into her time there. She was there to get to know the people, to experience the culture, to take up a completely new job, to further her already proficient knowledge of the Spanish language, and most of all, to enjoy herself. One dull dingy room wasn't going to make any difference. I felt instantly that we would get on well together but I had no idea then how very special a friend Sarah would become and how much we would be able to give to each other and help each other grow and develop during those nine months we shared a flat in Vigo.

Our most memorable drunken episode!

Life in Vigo took on a very different routine from the life we both had in England. Work would normally start at 10am each morning, except Mondays and Sundays, either teaching or preparing lessons. We would often eat breakfast and walk into school together, putting the world to rights and avoiding all the Vigo dog poo that seemed to line the pavements! Then we would usually come back to the flat for lunch and teach again from about 5.50 – 9.00 pm. By the end of the evening we were both usually too tired to prepare a meal at home so we often ate out and swilled everything down with a few beers and some dodgy cheap wine.

I remember one evening when Sarah and I were in particularly good spirits and the alcohol had been going down rather too well. We returned to the flat through the old part of Vigo, singing all the 70s and 80s pop songs that we could remember. Having some sensitivity and enough awareness that our neighbours may not appreciate our beautiful drunken singing, we stopped on arriving at our block of flats and then happily carried on once inside.

In the kitchen we drank coffee and ate toast, singing old Alison Moyet songs and songs from 'Grease' at the top of our voices, putting everything into it and hamming it up like real pop stars. Suddenly there was the slamming of about three doors and windows in the flat. We had totally forgotten that Frances, our other flat mate, was having a quiet night in with her boy friend who was over from England. Not only were the internal doors leading down the corridor to Frances's room open, but so too was the kitchen window that opened on to the inner courtyard. It appeared that we had been singing to at least ten other open windows at two in the morning!

Dancing

One of our favourite weekend haunts was the local Salsa club. Sarah and I both loved dancing and letting our hair down and this club hidden in the depths of old town Vigo was a real find.

At midnight the place suddenly came alive, filled with good-looking men who really knew how to swing their hips in the Latin American way! The best part about it as far as Sarah and I were concerned was that everyone there genuinely seemed to want to dance. The dance floor was always packed and there was none of the cattle market feel that was always the case in England. For me, dancing salsa was a completely new experience but as long as I had a strong partner to throw me around I could generally follow quite well. Without a decent partner I was hopeless! After going to this club a few times we realised that there seemed to be a hierarchy of dancers within the club. The best dancers picked only the best (or the best looking) dancers to dance with, and Sarah and I chuckled at the unspoken subtle politics that went on.

One character we found particularly amusing was a tall dark-haired man who was an excellent dancer but really knew it, and strutted around the place like a proud peacock. To add to our amusement he wore heeled boots and tight groin-hugging black trousers with an open-necked white shirt, allowing him to proudly show off his incredibly hairy chest and gleaming gold medallion. He obviously thought that anyone else he chose to dance with was truly honoured and he would raise his arms in the air, click his fingers and point at his next 'chosen one '.

So when his 'chosen one' was Sarah (and not on one occasion only) we both knew that she had reached the pinnacle of her salsa dancing career. Just to add to the humour of the situation, I was always asked to dance by an ageing, bald, beer-bellied, overweight gentleman with a sweaty brow and armpits. Sarah and I had many a laugh over who had the best or the worst deal that night!

Learning Spanish

When I accepted the job in Vigo, I was told that Spanish lessons would be included, which was very important to me as it was a language that I had never spoken before. A few weeks after we arrived, however, it became clear that no Spanish lessons had been organised for us.

We took up the matter with my boss, who decided that the best solution was for Sarah – a very proficient Spanish speaker – to teach myself and one other teacher in the same situation. Poor Sarah. She had expected to be teaching English to the Spanish, not Spanish to the English!

As the weeks went by it became clear that learning Spanish was never going to be my forte and of course when there was a choice between learning my Spanish verbs and going out for a meal, the latter always won! Sarah remained as patient as ever, never complained, and never laughed at my valiant attempt to communicate with the local shopkeepers. Sarah made a great effort to meet and

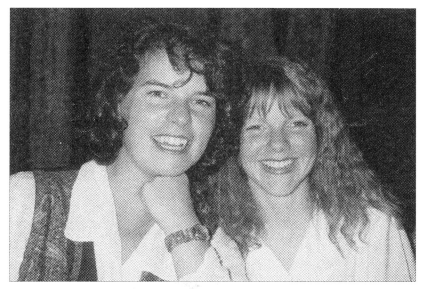

Andrea and Sarah in Vigo, Spring 1994

chat with the locals and I could always see the relief on their faces when they saw me walk into their shop accompanied by Sarah. Without her they knew that they had a lengthy language struggle on their hands.

I don't think Sarah ever felt that I was making any particular progress with my Spanish until the day I had an argument with José, a Spanish lad who shared our flat. Sarah and I would often make lunch in the flat together and we enjoyed the chance to eat in peace and quiet and get away from work for a few hours and inevitably moan about our boss, who at one point seemed to take great pleasure in making my life miserable. José was a student at the city university, so more often than not he was either at college or locked away in his room studying. For a couple of weeks he started to join us in the kitchen at lunchtime, and although he would never share our meals, preferring to cook his own, Sarah and I both saw this as an opportunity to speak Spanish with him and get to know him a little better.

But José had other plans. All his cooking was fried in deep olive oil which spat everywhere and smoked us out and José just wanted to watch the day-time quiz shows on the TV in the kitchen at full volume. Not only was he mono-syllabic in response to our questions, but Sarah and I could hardly speak to each other because the TV was so loud. After about a week of this I finally snapped and in my best Spanish I proceeded to have a heated dis-cussion about the volume of the TV. Sarah kept well out of the argument and looked on in amuse-ment at how I was managing to hold my own in a lan-guage that we had decided I was never

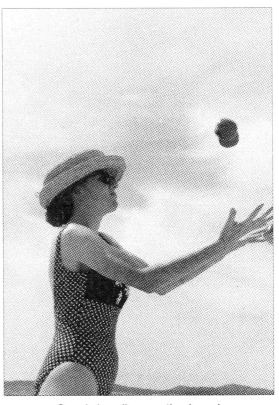

Sarah juggling on the beach

going to master! José was so stunned that I had challenged him at all, let alone in Spanish, that he turned the TV off and ate in his room. Whilst feeling guilty that he couldn't share the kitchen with us, I was amazed that I had managed to converse with him. We never had the problem with the TV again!

Steve's Arrival

As the weeks went by Sarah and I became great friends, and we spent a lot of time talking about our families and past relation-ships and both gave each other support over different aspects of our lives – usually concerning men!

I had met Steve just a few months before leaving for Spain and

I slowly came to realise while I was living abroad that perhaps he was a man I shouldn't allow to slip through my fingers. Sarah was supportive in many ways and often listened to my tales of woe and how much I missed him. She never seemed to mind the fact that she was sharing a flat with someone who really wanted to be in England and I like to think that Sarah took support from me when she needed it.

One example of Sarah's true dedication as a friend was when Steve was due to visit me for the Festival in February. As far as I was concerned, Steve was arriving on the Saturday and I had planned the week prior to his arrival in terms of work, socialising, cleaning the flat (my room particularly!) and finalising last details with Steve so I could meet him at the airport.

Unknown to me, Steve had arranged to surprise me by arriving a day early. He had sorted out all the details with Sarah. She had managed to jump to the phone every time it rang and bluff her way through conversations with Steve, pretending it was a friend when in fact she was making sure what time to expect him, giving him instructions and details on where to go and how to get there. She had also informed the remaining eight teachers at work about what was happening so they could all be waiting in the café with me after work when he arrived. To top the lot Sarah did an extra journey from school between two of her classes, back to the flat just to tidy up my room for me. She knew I was intending to make sure it was all spick and span the following day, and that the room looked as if a bomb had hit it on the day that Steve was due, so she prepared her lessons in double quick time and strode out the twenty-minute walk each way to clear the room up before he came. I could have kissed her!

Thanks to Sarah the grand arrival went according to plan. We had all finished work for the evening and were sitting down in the cafe, winding down and having a beer. Everyone knew Steve was arriving; except for me. On cue, he stumbled through the door, laden down with luggage, to a round of applause that seemed to come from everyone in the café. My face was a picture and all I could say was that my room was a tip and I was wearing the wrong underwear! A true friend indeed!

Our Flat

Although our flat was well-equipped, comfortable and only a short walk from the school, its biggest drawback was that it was very dark. My room overlooked a fairly busy road with noisy buses pulling up the hill. Sarah's room looked on to a dingy courtyard. Between morning and evening lessons we would often go for a walk down to the old harbour to soak up the sunshine and have a coffee or a glass of wine. If the weather was bad we would sit and chat in the kitchen or relax in our rooms while I would often write to Steve. When we first arrived in Vigo the weather was awful. It hardly ever seemed to stop raining, which made our flat seem even darker.

One day when I was sitting quietly in my room, missing Steve and wishing for better weather, a beautiful voice started to sing. At first I thought it was the radio or a neighbour, then I realised it was Sarah, singing her heart out in her small dingy room. She was not concerned by the closeness of all the other flats that looked on to the courtyard. And why not, when her singing was so beautiful?

The Death of Sarah's Dad

Our happy sunny days in Vigo came to an abrupt end one week before we were all due to fly home in June 1994. It had been a really hot day and a group of us had spent it at the local beach just playing around and soaking up the sun in an attempt to top up our tans before returning home. Our good mood continued into the evening so we ate out and then went on to a club. Sarah was having a great time socialising with some of the students that she had got to know quite well over the year.

By midnight I was pooped and decided to head home but Sarah was still firing on all cylinders and had decided to stay out a bit longer. I had returned to the flat and was just falling into bed when there was a knock on my door. It was Frances, looking as white as a sheet, and quite distressed. She told me that she had taken a call from Sarah's Mum who had phoned to say that Sarah's Dad had passed away as a result of a heart attack that evening.

I couldn't believe what I was hearing. I had never met Sarah's father but I felt as if I knew him through Sarah and the long conversations we had had about our families. Sarah always spoke with such pride and love about all her family and I could tell she had a huge amount of respect for her father. Almost immediately I felt the huge loss for Sarah and her family and then I realised that we were going to have to break this terrible news to her. How on earth do you break such devastating news to your closest friend?

Poor Val phoned a few times before Sarah returned to the flat. Frances was actually on the phone to Val when Sarah walked through the door. At least Sarah could hear the news from her own Mum. Of course there was nothing Frances or I could do except hold Sarah and be there with her.

That night seemed to last for ever. We all stayed up together helping Sarah pack. Once Sarah had got over the initial shock she went into auto pilot. She seemed so calm and practical.

* * *

By June 1994 Bruce Hotter was Managing Director of Barclay's Bank Computer Operations, based at Radbroke Hall near Knutsford. On the evening of June 12th, Bruce died suddenly during a convivial evening with Val and some friends. From the hospital in the early morning Val telephoned Sarah who was in Vigo, Spain, and Mark, who was in Weston super Mare. Sarah arrived at Manchester Airport by that afternoon. Mark and his girl friend Sarah were at the home of Sarah's aunt. By six in the morning they were with Val.

Extracts from the Address by family friend John Mulholland at the Mass in Thanksgiving for the Life of Bruce John Hotter, held at St Vincent's RC Church, Altrincham, on 21 June 1994:

"The great numbers in church today are eloquent testimony to the love and admiration we all had for Bruce.

"While still a toddler, Bruce had those twinkling eyes and that engaging smile that were so much a part of him. His eleven years at sea brought him great satisfaction, never more so than when he met Valerie, a passenger on one of his ships. Valerie's return ticket remained unused.

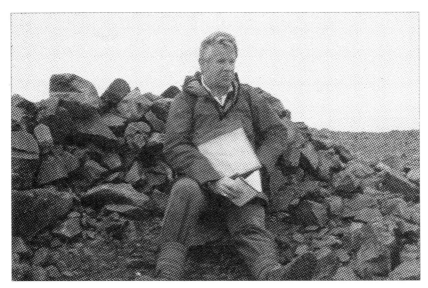

Bruce – with his faithful copy of 'Wainwright'

"When Bruce, engaged to Valerie, returned to Argentina, those eyes and that smile instantly won over Valerie's parents at their very first meeting with him – even more so than the excellent buffet which Bruce provided for them on the ship.

"Much as he loved the sea, Bruce decided, when Sarah was expected, that the place to be was at home with his family. He joined Barclay's Bank, becoming Managing Director of Computer Operations. His colleagues remember his respect for people, his interest in their opinions, his natural charm, and, despite all his achievements, his unassuming character.

"Bruce's *joie de vivre* was infectious. Whether walking the Lakeland Fells, or sailing his boat, or sharing a meal and good wine, or listening to music, or playing party games (and don't we remember those Hotter parties!), or enjoying conversation, all of us were enriched by being with him.

"It was in his own family, of Valerie, Sarah and Mark that Bruce was most fulfilled and gave the very best of himself. His deep love and pride in his children was evident to us all. Much though he loved a sing-song round the piano, singing was not his greatest talent. But he managed to send Sarah and Mark to sleep with lullabies which showed great inventiveness. A challenge which he rose to less successfully was that of trying to get a word in edgeways when Valerie and Sarah were speaking!

"Of course we are all grieving at this time. But grief must not be our prevailing feeling, for good reasons. Firstly, we can be thankful for Bruce's life, for the strength as well as the gentleness, for the breadth of vision as well as the care for detail. Secondly, the Christian faith which brings us together today proclaims the hope of the Resurrection and of a life to come in which we shall all know our loved ones again. Thirdly, Bruce would not wish us – does not wish us – to go on grieving but to remember the blessings, the joys, the laughter and the love.

"Last Christmas, as St Paul put it in that wonderful passage from Corinthians which Sarah read so beautifully earlier in the Mass, Bruce saw 'a dim reflection in a mirror', but now he sees 'face to face'. Next Christmas, we may be sure, the celebration of the Nativity in heaven will be joined by Bruce's twinkling eyes and his engaging smile."

*   *   *

In a note attached to her copy of this Oration, Val says:" So much of what John says about Bruce's character and what made him a likeable person, you could also say of Sarah and Mark."

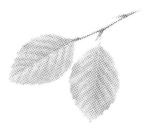

Chapter 8
THE SALT MUSEUM
1996 – 1998

There are no days in life so memorable
as those which vibrated to some stroke of the imagination

R. W. Emerson, ' Beauty ', The Conduct of Life, 1860

SARAH was appointed Community and Education Officer of the Salt Museum in Northwich in January 1996.

When I visited the museum to talk to some of her former colleagues in the education department, I was treated to tea served in elegant colourful cups, with a plate of equally colourful cakes. Just like the "old" days, I was told; Sarah was very fond of cake and biscuits!

At the museum I met Ann O'Brien, Valda MacDonald, Carol Booth and Shirley Starkey who all worked with Sarah in the museum's Education Department. They remember that Sarah came across as a very capable person, who obviously loved her job. She was comfortable and relaxed, straightforward and to the point. She was skilled at interviewing and talking to people, without "grilling them". She valued her staff's opinions. Once, when some very young children were about to arrive, she said: "Do you want to do the babbies this morning?" The staff remember her smilingly, and with affection.

Carol affirmed that Sarah was the ideal boss because she was a fair person, and "as lovely with the children as with the rest of

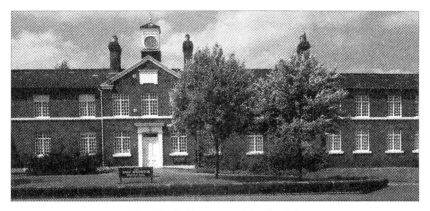

The Salt Museum, Northwich

SALT has been produced in Cheshire for over two thousand years and it is the only place in Britain where it is still produced on a large scale. The Salt Museum tells the fascinating story of mid-Cheshire and the industry that has shaped the landscape and the lives of those who live there. There has been a Salt Museum in Northwich for over a hundred years. It began in the library in the town centre and moved into Weaver Hall in 1981. The Museum is administered by Cheshire County Council. The education services provide taught sessions and resources for schools and other groups on a wide range of topics, from a day in the life of a Victorian salt worker, to the natural and the industrial environment, and to the Romans. There is also an exciting programme of events during the holidays and weekends.

us". Everything Sarah did seemed to come naturally to her – "she just touched everything the right way." The shared lunches and chats in the kitchen are fondly remembered by the staff. "It was a joy to eat and talk with her." Sarah was not a Tupperware person; she would bring an ordinary lunch bag. It usually contained yoghurt, and a good supply of biscuits and cake. They recall with awe the way that Sarah peeled, sectioned and relished an orange.

A Day in the Life ...
Of Community & Education Officer, Sarah Hotter

Sarah is based at the Salt Museum, Northwich, and has responsibility for community and education activities there and at Stretton Watermill, near Farndon. She has been in the post since January 1996.

9.00am Arrive at the Museum at the same time as a costume maker with replica Victorian costume for the new Victorian Miller school session at Stretton. Have to try on the gorgeous pink bonnets. Not really my colour.

9.15am Today is a catching up day as there are no school or other parties visiting the museum. Calls include:
• Organising a meeting with the Hallé Orchestra's Gamelan Co-ordinator as we will be having a "Gamelan in the Galleries Week" in the autumn. (A gamelan is a set of Javanese percussion instruments).
• Advising a school on doing an archaeological dig
• Chatting to a local TEC about a teacher's work for the Stretton education pack

11.00am Meet a local craftsperson to plan the half-term workshop, "Huge, Sticky Paintings".

12.00 noon A high school teacher drops in unexpectedly. Some 'A'-level pupils want to produce an audio guide for the Museum for the visually impaired. Can I help? You bet!

12.30pm Over lunch, the attendant and I discuss what visitor information we can get from our newly souped-up till.

1.45pm Tim, who has learning disabilities, arrives for his weekly afternoon of work experience. I set him to work on stuffing envelopes with the new Stretton leaflets to schools. He seems to be settling in well and enjoying work here.

2.00-3.00pm Finally a bit of time to write out the script for the new Victorian Miller session. The first guinea pig school will experience life 1874 mill-style next week, so fingers crossed. The stuffed mice I ordered still haven't arrived... Must phone the supplier.

3.00-4.00pm Write out booking forms for visiting groups to both sites and prepare for the interviews for the new miller.

4.00pm Helen, a high school student, visits to chat about her two weeks work placement starting next week.

5.00pm Think about moving a few boxes of education material that need carrying up from the cellar, but decide tomorrow will do. Time for home. Hope I'm ahead of the football traffic on my way back to Manchester.

(From Community Matters, edited by Rose Kilfoyle and Di Hanning-Lee, Community Police. Telephone 01244 602182/2102)

To them, this performance was an art form!

Sarah's former colleagues at the Salt Museum all agree that the department prospered under her leadership. Bookings from schools and other groups increased, and the staff attribute this to Sarah's positivity and her ability to create a very immediate rapport with people. She had her clear ideas and objectives, but was always keen to hear other people's ideas and to act on them when appropriate. Sarah could sound very authoritative if she had to, but mostly she was quiet, gentle and jokey. In meetings she was very clear in the way she could explain things. When Sarah was quite ill she organised a major educational event at Manchester Airport, and course members rang afterwards to say how good it was.

From her appointment in 1996, to the spring of 1998 when she was taken ill, Sarah appeared fine. In the words of Carol, she "effervesced". But by the time Sarah set off with Val for their holiday in Ireland, Carol had noticed that Sarah was "out of sync" on more than one occasion when greeting the arriving group of children and explaining to them the order of activities for the day. At the time these small slips could be passed off as tiredness.

Carol's daughter is called Sarah, and the same age. Carol often thinks of Sarah Hotter, and tries to imagine herself in Val's position. She thinks how brave Val and Sarah were as Sarah's condition worsened; she considers it "unbelievable" how they faced up to the situation. "They are such a close family; it came across in everything Sarah said about her Mum, her Dad and her brother. They were lovely, all of them."

Valda enjoyed her lunchtime chats with Sarah. Sarah told Valda how much she enjoyed her "girlie" weekends, doing exciting things with Val. The two had been to the turkish baths at Harrogate, and Sarah liked to visit her brother Mark at High Wycombe. Valda notes Sarah's communication skills, her sense of fairness, and her modesty. Many would have let it be known that they were an Oxford graduate, but Sarah did not; she might just mention, in general terms "when I was at College..."

At the museum I happened to meet Carol's mother. She told me about fond recollections of Sarah by the members of the Northwich Inner Wheel Ladies Group. When the group visited

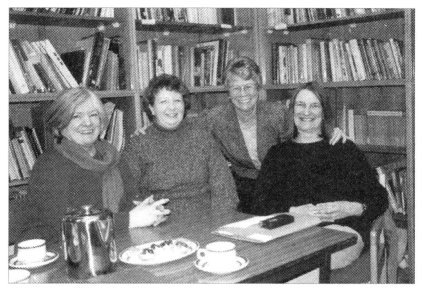

L-R: Shirley, Valda, Anne and Carol

the Salt Museum, Sarah was so pleased with the things they told her about the old times in Northwich. Everyone commented afterwards on how pleasant Sarah was, and they kept in touch with her during her illness.

The staff were struck by Sarah's acceptance of her condition when she returned to the Museum after the Ireland holiday. At first, apart from the occasional memory lapse there was no outward sign that she was ill. Later, Sarah had hair loss caused by chemotherapy, and took to wearing a black cloche hat. She continued working as much as she could; she kept up her treatment sessions, and she attended Spanish classes at night school. To her staff, her demeanour was utterly relaxed and confident. As the illness took hold, Sarah eventually attended personal therapy sessions. But still, say the staff, she was helping them at least as much as they were trying to help and protect her. Anne remembers the staff Christmas meal in 1998. Sarah was keen to enjoy the occasion with her colleagues. She was in a merry mood and ate heartily.

After Sarah's diagnosis, and the surgery which followed swiftly afterwards, she continued to work as much as she could.

Because she could no longer drive after spring 1998, Sarah travelled by train to Northwich and back from her home in Hale, a pleasant journey across the Cheshire countryside. The Museum staff would collect her at Northwich station, then return her there. At Hale, Val would be waiting; she recalls Sarah walking over the footbridge in her brown coat and matching hat.

At work, Sarah did what she could. If she had to be absent, Val would ring to keep the Museum colleagues informed about Sarah's condition. Sarah did not hide the truth; she shared it with her staff.

Anne is sure that Sarah had "a faith to hang on to", and she envies her for it. She is sure that without this faith, the story of Sarah would have been very different. Anne says Sarah never gave in to her illness. She always saw a light at the end of the tunnel, and it was so obvious that she was not going to be beaten. Even when her illness was well advanced, Sarah mentioned a new treatment that had been offered. "I've nothing to lose, so I'll try it anyway."

The Museum staff knew Sarah did have bad days, but were sure she was never afraid of dying because, as she told them herself, she knew death was not the end, and that she would enter into eternal life. Anne attended Sarah's funeral, and describes it as "a wonderful service; what everyone would aim to achieve".

Spiritual matters were part of the lunchtime conversations. Shirley sold Traidcraft products, to help workers in underdeveloped countries. Sarah was very keen to improve the plight of such people, and she thought it would be good to have only Traidcraft coffee for her staff to drink. But this product was not the favourite flavour at the Salt Museum, and the staff think the huge tin of it is probably still on top of a cupboard!

Sarah's personal faith was noted also by Shirley, who said: "I am sure it gave her strength. I saw it in her attitude to life and the easy way she could talk about The Lord."

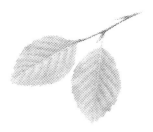

Chapter 9
HOPE AND CHRISTIE'S
1998 – 1999

However broken down is the spirit's shrine,
the spirit is there all the time

Nigerian Proverb

IN the spring of 1998 Sarah was working hard at the Salt Museum. She and Val decided to have a holiday in Ireland. The plan was to fly to Cork, where they would hire a car to explore the far south west of Ireland.

At Manchester Airport Val looked askance at their small aircraft. As they climbed the steps, Val wondered if she would make it to Cork, or if she would be ill on the flight. She told Sarah that if she saw sellotape anywhere on the plane she would not get on it. The journey passed without incident. At Cork Sarah collected their car and drove herself and Val to the hotel. It would be the last time that Sarah drove a car. That evening the two enjoyed a meal at a lovely restaurant.

For breakfast the next morning, Sarah and Val shared a table with some other guests.

Sarah rubbed her side, shuddered, and told Val she felt funny. She tried to carry on with her breakfast, but then left the table. Val followed. In her room Sarah said she felt pins and needles up and down her right hand side. Val requested a doctor, and the hotel called one who was on weekend stand-by duty.

The doctor carried out a thorough examination, and it was obvious to Val that he was testing Sarah neurologically. The doctor requested a scan, and Sarah was taken in the hotel minibus to the Mercy Hospital in Cork, run by the Sisters of Mercy. She was admitted to the Accident and Emergency Department, immediately made comfortable in a bed and examined separately by two more doctors.

The following morning the first scan was taken, but the image was not clear enough and a marker was injected. The second scan took place that afternoon. Sarah phoned Val in great distress to report than an abnormality had been found. The hospital advised Val and Sarah to return home immediately to see their GP and consult a neurosurgeon without delay. So the holiday was abandoned and Val and Sarah took the next flight home. They saw their GP the next day, and on the day after that Sarah was seen by Mr James Leggate, Consultant Neurosurgeon at the Hope Hospital in Salford, Manchester.

Less than a week later, Sarah was operated on by Mr Leggate. Val and Mark were with her on the morning of the operation. Sarah, brisk and breezy, was watching Breakfast TV. A "pre-med" was offered, to relax her and make her drowsy before she went to theatre, but she declined it, pointing out that Breakfast TV is enough to drive anyone to sleep. As she was wheeled off on the trolley, Val said, "Give them hell, Sarah, and no swearing at the doctors in Spanish." Sarah went off laughing and chatting.

THE PATIENT, THE PERSON
James Leggate, Consultant Neurosurgeon, Hope Hospital, Salford:

"I was first contacted about Sarah when her GP phoned me on the 28th May asking me if I could see one of his patients who had just had her 32nd birthday and who whilst on holiday in Cork had been admitted to hospital there. Investigations had suggested the presence of a brain tumour.

"Sarah came the following day with her mother to see me in my office at Hope Hospital. By that stage I had a clearer picture of the results of her tests in Ireland, following a fax giving me the results

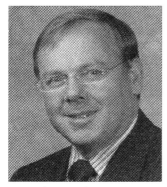

James Leggate

of tests carried out at the Mercy Hospital in Cork.

"Sarah's history was a very short one. She had developed some headaches three or four weeks previously but had not thought much about these at the time. She described how she had initially had some pins and needles in the right arm and leg, which had started two weeks earlier. Five days before seeing me she had noticed that these tingling pins and needles sensations had failed to settle as they normally did. Sarah was sufficiently distressed to call a doctor in Cork to see her in the hotel where she was staying.

"After seeing the doctor Sarah was referred to the Accident and Emergency Unit at the Mercy Hospital in Cork, and subsequently returned to the United Kingdom, having had to cut short her holiday.

"When I asked Sarah and her mother into my office it was quite apparent that they were close. During our initial conversation I was struck by how much strength they were able to draw not only from each other but from within themselves at such a stressful time. Sarah was able to take in the news that I was giving her and the impact that this was likely to have on her life.

"Initially I felt the best thing for Sarah was to obtain a diagnosis and I put this to her as the next step in managing her illness. Sarah did not merely accept what I was saying but rather, without challenging, was able to question the options available to her which we then discussed, before she made the decision as to how she wished to go forward. Sarah's attitude throughout my early meeting with her was one of confidence. Confidence in her ability within her family to get through this life-changing event, and confidence in those around her and involved in her care to look after her.

"After some further tests Sarah was admitted to Hope Hospital in early June 1998 and underwent a computer-guided stereotactic craniotomy and biopsy of her tumour. Post-operatively she remained well, but unfortunately the results of the tissue examination showed that this was a highly malignant tumour, arising within the brain tissue itself.

"I had a long talk with Sarah and her mother and at that time Sarah felt that she wanted to know the details of the treatment options that were available to her, but neither she nor her mother at that stage wished to discuss in great detail the prognosis. I remember Sarah saying to me, and this was agreed with her mother, that she would prefer to take it one step at a time. This approach was one that I fully appreciated and could feel comfortable with, so we moved to the next stage in her short illness, which was to invite the staff from the Christie Hospital to consider Sarah for further treatment, either in the form of radiotherapy or chemotherapy, or a combination of the two.

"Having been seen in the middle of June at the Hope Hospital by the Christie Hospital staff Sarah was allowed home to begin her radiotherapy, which she finished in mid-July. Her chemotherapy ran for six weeks from the end of July. I next saw Sarah in November when I found her to be as positive as ever. Once again Sarah, her mother and myself all sat down and discussed the treatment options that I had already raised with her, and in addition other treatments which she had heard about both through friends and contacts, as well as on the Internet.

"Once again I was struck with Sarah's ability to explore all the avenues that were available to her without in the least way challenging those people in whom she had placed her trust and her confidence to best manage her illness. We had long discussions about the experimental treatments that were being tried in various units, together with the variety of alternative treatments that were on offer. I was aware however that Sarah, whilst happy to discuss the various options, was beginning to develop an inner peace, an acceptance that was beginning to prepare her for the time when she would acknowledge that despite all our best endeavours her disease would inevitably progress. In no way however did this development of an inner peace and an ability to accept her lot, leave Sarah gloomy. She got frustrated at times and this was mainly because of the effects on her speech which the tumour was exerting. As someone who had always been eloquent and relied strongly on her spoken word to communicate with people around her, this for Sarah, was, I think, one of the hardest things to come to terms with.

"Sadly the tumour progressed, despite her chemotherapy and radiotherapy and in early 1999 Sarah began to develop recurrent symptoms, which indicated the tumour was growing again. She was admitted in April 1999 to the neurosurgical unit, where we discussed the return of her tumour and the fact that this had now grown quite considerably in size. I explained that further surgery could limit the pressure effects that the tumour was beginning to exert on the surrounding brain but I was quite honest to Sarah and her family and explained that this would not alter the ulti-mate outcome of this tumour's progression. Nevertheless, as a way of improving the quality of her life, in someone who was so young and so vital, and who had so many things that she still wanted to do and achieve, we, all of us, felt that further surgery was the right course to take. Sarah therefore came into theatre on 28th April 1999, knowing that this last operation would give her some extra months but also understanding and accepting that it would not affect the ultimate outcome. I remember her in theatre before we put her to sleep for her last operation smiling and jok-ing with the anaesthetist and myself over the fact that having lost her lovely head of hair with the radiotherapy, the need to avoid a head shave was really not relevant.

"After the operation Sarah had some slight problems with her speech but this soon settled and before she went home Sarah, her mother and I sat down and discussed the implications of the tumour's recurrence, and where we would go from now. Once again I found them very supportive of each other, each drawing strength not only from each other but from that unfathomable source which no one can identify but which exists for all human beings when they are in times of difficulty, whether that difficulty be illness, stress, hurt or grief. For those people with a faith this strength comes from God but for others it is a powerful force which they know they can reach out and rely upon. Sarah and her mother both had a strong faith. As a family they had already had their faith tested before Sarah's illness began. The quiet confi-dence and growing inner peace within Sarah was becoming much more obvious to those around her and to those who were looking after her.

"Her cheeky optimism remained, and further chemotherapy began soon after Sarah's second operation. Sadly, her condition deteriorated and as we know from other aspects in this book more people became involved in her care in the last months of her life.

"I have no doubt that this young lady will have left her mark on the lives of these people in the same way as she left her mark on mine. I would hope that if by reading this story others in similar circumstances will be able to draw strength from Sarah's example, then her life and all that came from it, including this book, will not only have been worthwhile but will have been a justification for this young spirit's inclusion in our world."

'DOCTOR WOW' - Dr H Rao Gattamaneni

Following her treatment at Hope Hospital, Sarah was referred to the care of the Christie Hospital, the specialist centre for cancer

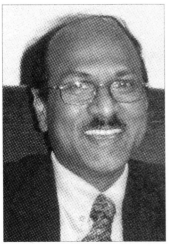

patients in the Manchester area. Known to his younger patients as "Dr Wow", Dr H Rao Gattamaneni *(pictured left)* has been Consultant Clinical Oncologist at the Christie since 1978.

Oncology is the management of patients with cancers. Dr Rao's special interests are patients with brain tumours – as in Sarah's case – and younger patients with various types of cancer.

A sensitive unassuming man from Andra Pradesh in eastern India, Dr Rao formed an early interest in cancer during his undergraduate medical studies. One of his textbooks had been written by a consultant at the Christie. Dr Rao undertook specialist post-graduate studies in India, then came to the Christie in 1976 for two years' study of the latest oncological techniques. He is still there!

When Dr Rao first saw Sarah at the Christie in 1998, they both knew she had a life-threatening tumour. To Dr Rao, Sarah came

THE CHRISTIE HOSPITAL
Wilmslow Road, Withington, Manchester

Christie's, located a few miles south of Manchester city centre, began in 1892 as a home for people with cancer. The money came from a fortune left for the people of Manchester by the industrialist Sir Joseph Whitworth.

In 1901 the home was renamed the Christie Hospital in honour of estate trustee Chancellor Richard Copley Christie and his wife Helen, a driving force in the development of the hospital. Confronted with new diseases such as mule spinner's cancer from the local cotton industry, and chimney sweep's cancer, doctors started looking for possible links to machine oils and airborne soot.

That early work was the forerunner of many breakthroughs made by researchers at Christie's.

Among the milestones are:

1901 use of Roentgen rays (X-rays) for therapy

1905 use of radium for therapy

1944 world's first clinical trial of a drug – used for breast cancer

1970 world's first clinical use of tamoxifen for breast cancer

1986 world's first use of cultured bone marrow for leukaemia treatment

1991 world's first single harvest blood stem-cell transplant

The Christie Hospital combined with the Holt Radium Institute in new premises opened on the present site in 1932. In the 1930s and onwards Dr Ralston Paterson built up a team of clinicians and physicians who turned the hospital into a world-renowned centre for the treatment of cancer by radiation. Dr Paterson's wife, Dr Edith Paterson, started research work at the Christie in 1938, initially alone, unpaid, and having to provide her own equipment. She too became a world-renowned pioneer in biological dosimetry, childhood cancers and anti-cancer drug treatment methods.

In 1966 new laboratories, bought by the Women's' Trust Fund, were opened. The laboratories, named the Paterson Institute for Cancer Research, are supported by the Cancer Research Campaign and remain world leaders.

Christie's Against Cancer marked the hospital's centenary in 2001 by raising £25 million for a linked series of projects identified by the Christie specialists as essential to enable the provision of the most modern, most innovative research and patient treatment facilities.

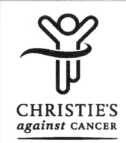

CHRISTIE'S
against CANCER

Real Help for Real Hope
Registered Charity No. 1049751

BRISTOL CANCER HELP CENTRE
0117 980 9500 info@bristolcancerhelp.org

Sarah and Val spent three days at the Bristol Centre. It opened in 1980 and is well known nationally for helping patients and their relatives to cope with cancer. It has a strong philosophy of comfort and spirituality in the non-religious sense. The aim is to eliminate negative thoughts and set a positive agenda tailored for individual needs. The activities – all optional – include talks by therapists, private healing sessions and discussions, music and some taught meditation. The Centre believes that those who react to cancer with a positive approach are more able to help themselves and use their positive spirit effectively.

Sarah and Val attended a full range of sessions, including "visualisation", a way of detaching the mind and transferring it to a pleasant place, like travelling on a magic carpet to a distant island. There were also discussions on dieting, and opportunities for private talks with doctors. Anyone can share feelings, in group or individual meetings. Without being under the illusion of a miracle cure, Val and Sarah found their visit very valuable emotionally and spiritually. The Centre provided much practical help for them. People supported each other. A large American lady presented Sarah with a bag of goodies from the Centre shop. Sarah was quite overcome by this spontaneous act of kindness, but her difficulties in speaking were increasing. Val was on hand to supply the words that Sarah could not find.

across initially as very anxious and probably angry, but also "a very determined lady who was not going to accept that nothing could be done". Notwithstanding her recent major brain surgery, Sarah was "very much with it". Sarah quizzed him closely about any treatment that might help her. She formed a comfortable relationship with Dr Rao, her medical consultant. They both looked forward to their future meetings.

Dr Rao recalls Sarah as being "always in the driving seat; very friendly, very cheerful, very straight, and very positive." Even during her final admission to the Christie, from 8-25 December 1999, she stayed in control to the end. Between periods of unconsciousness, she told the people with her "exactly what is what".

As Dr Rao puts it, "I am here to treat a person, an individual, not just a number. I can't go away and forget. With young people especially, we get involved, not just with the person's physical needs but also with their emotional needs, and the emotional needs of the family as well." Dr Rao deals with "wonderful bright lovely young people who would have a lot of life to live, but who are dying, beyond any further medical intervention we can provide; it is very distressing. Many parents fall apart. Lives are destroyed. The lives of siblings, and professional careers are affected."

Oncology is not without happier moments, but it is basically a very stressful occupation. This is especially so in the management of brain tumours, an area that many doctors prefer to avoid. Brain cancers are complex. Thought and speech patterns are affected, making it harder for the patient to communicate and make decisions.

When I visited the Christie it was teeming with people. The pressures on staff and patients must be immense, but every effort is made to ensure that the individual's needs are met. As soon as he has dealt with one patient, Dr Rao must focus on the next.

Sarah and Dr Rao became friends. She placed her trust in him, believing that in the long term things might get better. She tolerated the side effects of chemotherapy and was happy when her condition improved. When things became difficult again she remained very positive. Sarah kept her Plan of Action, and always had her questions ready for Dr Rao. Her attitude was "we can deal with this; let's get on with it". By being so methodical, Sarah helped Dr Rao to work with her. In her case, unlike many others, there was no need to use up precious time "beating around the bush".

Each Christmas morning Dr Rao remembers Sarah and her family. There is sadness, of course, for patients who die, but elation, too, for those who recover. Some former patients invite Dr Rao to their weddings, then bring their children to see him.

On Friday mornings Dr Rao runs a Late Effects Clinic for patients who have warded off cancer. He checks about twenty of them at a time, once or twice a year. He likes this way of ending his working week on a positive note. At home – close to the Christie for obvious reasons – Dr Rao enjoys time with his wife and daughter, his friends, and Indian films. He believes in a "greater power" which helps him in his work. Patients such as Sarah, though they may not survive, leave a lasting impression through the friendship formed through their illness. Other patients are luckier, and live out their natural lives. All patients have their positive aspects, and as Dr Rao points out, "It is the positive aspects that make me tick."

Val Hotter notes:
Sarah and I liked Dr Rao from the start and we grew to like him more and more as time went on. He established a non-fussy working relationship with Sarah and made it easy for us to feel comfortable with him. He dealt with her in a calm, kind, considerate, professional way, handling each situation as it presented itself and not crossing bridges before she felt ready for them. He is just the sort of doctor one wants on one's side in a crisis. Mark and I will always be grateful for his support, his gentleness and his kindness.

FOR SARAH

Epitaph from the tomb of Elizabeth Winkley, who died on 12 February 1756 and is buried at Bath Abbey:

> Her understanding was excellent
> Her genius innocently sprightly
> Her heart sincere and generous
> Her conversation agreeable
> Her friendship constant
> Her mind & person equally amiable

…. *"just like Sarah"*

From the hymn *For All The Saints*:

> …and when the strife is fierce
> The warfare long
> Steals on the ear the distant triumph-song
> And hearts are brave again
> and arms are strong…

Bishop W. Walsham How

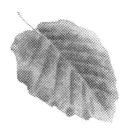

Chapter 10
RECOLLECTIONS

Memory is not so brilliant as hope
but it is more beautiful and a thousand times as true

George Dennison Prentice, 1860

THE DOLL
Ann Hotter, Sarah's aunt:
"Sarah was born in 1966 but I didn't meet her until she was two, as 1966 was the year that my parents came to visit me in Canada. However, I heard a lot about her, from her parents and particularly her grandparents and I received many pictures.

"Sarah was the first grandchild for my parents and the plump little red-head was adored by them. Once she started talking she and Grandpa would hold long conversations, including ones on tape to me. After a visit to Argentina with Valerie and Mark (I think she was about four and a half) she developed an Argentinian accent; at least it sounded that way to me on tape. Sarah had a beautiful singing voice; I think she inherited her chattiness and her musical abilities from her mother's side – it certainly wasn't from the Hotters.

"I liked to sew and I used to make little dresses and knit jumpers for Sarah. Valerie always made sure that pictures were taken of her and that I got copies. When I was a child I wanted a doll who could talk and walk and never received one, so I bought one for Sarah and made it a lot of clothes. I took it back with me, probably when she was four and I think it was a success. (Val told me that much later, when she was about thirteen, Sarah passed on the doll and its clothes, for other children to enjoy).

"I was in England in 1977 prior to Sarah's attendance at Grammar School and I went to the Open House for new pupils and parents with them. The new girls were required to have a particular edition of the Bible and a sex education book. Bruce dutifully bought both and when we returned to Arthog Road Sarah disappeared with the latter book, which she devoured (in true family fashion) in about an hour. She had already been told the "facts of life" by her parents but when she turned up in the kitchen with a question Bruce visibly braced himself. It turned out to be something quite innocuous but after she left we chuckled.

"Sarah visited me in 1982 on her own for four weeks after she took O-levels. She was the first person in her immediate family to visit here, apart from Bruce who had been here several times when he was in the Merchant Navy. (It was due to him that I ventured out here 'for two years' and stayed forever). Sarah was a delight to have as a visitor. To me, one of her strongest attributes became obvious then and for the rest of her life. This was the ability to become involved in everything new that was on offer, even if it was perhaps something that didn't particularly appeal to her and which she might never do again; she made the most of every experience of life that presented itself. One aspect of this was that she *listened* to what people were saying and was concerned about other people. My husband Cliff Rundgren (who was my boyfriend in 1982) particularly remembers two conversations with her. One was about Labour History (Cliff's great interest) in which Sarah showed a lot of interest and knowledge. The other concerned the differences in accent and pronunciation (UK, Canada, USA etc). Sarah had the ability, unconscious, I think, of picking up and copying accents.

"One slight exception to the 'try anything once' aspect was on a trip to Seattle. We did the sights and then went for dinner in a family seafood restaurant. The first part of the meal was a 'bucket of clams'. Sarah, after much thought ate one! I ate about five and Cliff ate the rest.

"We went over to Vancouver Island by ferry and stayed with a friend in Victoria, the capital of the province of British Columbia. It is a delightful city, very "British" at that point, with a lot of beautiful scenery and interesting sights, including the Provincial Museum.

"Our main trip was a camping trip was to the Rockies; a must for every tourist. Camping in North America is very different from Guide camps. There are beautiful individual campsites, often in forests, with picnic tables and seats and campfires with wood provided. Sometimes there are even bears, although we didn't have any. Sarah helped cook meals and we had a great time. We went for a lot of hikes in the mountains. Sub-alpine meadows full of flowers are one of the glories of North America. We also saw mountain sheep, mountain goats, marmots, squirrels, deer. The Banff to Jasper highway is one of the most beautiful in the world and we were there before it got too full of tourist buses.

"Another memorable day trip from Vancouver was a hike in the Mt Baker area of Washington State. Mt Baker is a volcanic peak over 10,000 feet high, the most northerly of the string of peaks that go down into California. Mt. St. Helen's is in the middle. This hike was memorable not just for the view of Mt. Baker and the flowers but for the blackflies. The flies 'liked' Sarah even better than me and we ate lunch with our parkas on, hoods up, stuffing sandwiches into our mouths. Then we left!

"In July 1987 I stayed with Sarah in Oxford for her last two nights there. She was still in her student flat and must have been in her vegetarian phase as she cooked pasta with pinenuts for dinner. We spent a whole day visiting 'her' Oxford. I had lived in Cambridge for several years so I knew that city and university well and it was interesting to see the differences and the similarities.

"Later on Cliff and I had two of our most enjoyable holidays ever with the family. One was a marvellous week of eating, drinking and walking in the Lake District on the occasion of Bruce and Valerie's silver wedding in May 1989. I remember her walking alongside Bruce, hand tucked into his bent arm, chattering away. The other was the Christmas that we spent in Hale with them all. It was a time of happiness and laughter."

A SPECIAL NOISY LAUGH
Vanesa Cabaña, Sarah's cousin in Argentina:

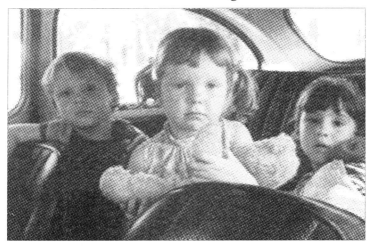

Sarah NOT smiling! With cousin Richard, left, and cousin Vanesa.

"I really don't know where to start with my stories about Sarah since her first trip to Argentina.

"In Cordoba, when we were quite small, she always slept with her Teddy bear. Wherever she went she always carried her special little friend.

"When we were about nine, around 1975, the Hotters came to Buenos Aires to spend Christmas and New Year with us. I will never forget that Christmas. On Christmas Eve Norman, Mark, Richard, Sarah and I couldn't sleep; we were so excited.

"We were all gathered together, in the dark, in the upstairs hall which leads to the bedrooms, looking out of the windows on to the garden. We were talking excitedly till my mother came up to tell us to go to bed as it was very late.

"The following morning we saw some improvised Christmas stockings hanging off the ends of our beds. They were made out of ladies' stockings and you could see the little presents poking out of the tops. For us Argentines this was an entirely new experience because Christmas stockings are not a tradition in Argentina as they are in European countries. We woke up early to gather down stairs around the huge Christmas tree.

"I remember thinking that never in my childhood had I seen a tree like it, surrounded by all the presents. It was a more than beautiful Christmas.

"On another occasion during this trip we were driving along the coast road bordering the River Plate, Argentina's principal river, and I remember that Bruce and Val asked my father to stop in front of one of the many stalls. They were selling watermelons, melons and all different types of fruit. The size, colour and quantity of fruit being sold surprised not only Bruce but also Sarah and Mark.

"In Buenos Aires we visited San Martin Square on a very hot afternoon. The grown-ups took refuge under the trees while we youngsters played hide and seek amongst the Palos Borrachos, magnolias and jacarandas. We also played Pin and Poy, a game using a plastic rugby-shaped ball with a perforated middle, strung on long cords and whizzed to and fro between two players. We spent many hours playing in the sun and in the end we all took off our clothes and played in our 'undies'. At first Sarah refused to take off her dress and I imitated her because I regarded her as older, despite the small difference in our ages. She was always the taller of the two. Finally our mothers persuaded us and we took off our dresses.

"Sarah was a little girl who suffered a lot from the heat and the sun. We really loved being out in the fresh air, and swimming. Sarah always had to put on a strong factor sun cream and hardly ever took off her T shirt; her skin was so white. I remember how we escaped to Maria's little kiosk, a typical Argentine hole-in-the-wall sweets/newspapers/drinks stall, to ask for water ice creams and other sweets. Maria would give us some sweet or other, on condition we would say nothing about it!.

"Sarah always stood out because of the paleness of her skin and the colour of her hair. Everyone noticed. When she was older, Sarah 'the red head' (the family always referred to her as *'la colorada'*) would spend quite some time during the day brushing her hair. She always looked spotless. She loved reading and would bring a couple of books on each trip out to us. When anyone asked after Sarah and couldn't see her, I would tell them that she must be upstairs in the bedroom reading her book, and there she would be, sitting or lying, enjoying her reading."

Val writes: "When Sarah was quite little, Bruce adopted the pet name 'my little sausage' for her. The word 'sausage' stuck and she was often called that. Being a good Argentine, I translated it into Spanish, *salchicha*, and the first part of the word *salchi* also stuck. She would readily answer to 'Salchi'. I remember that on one occasion a business colleague of Bruce's took him, Sarah and me out to dinner. I was telling him this story – the *salchi* one – and he didn't believe me. So I called out to Sarah, who was putting her face on upstairs: 'Salchi!' She answered immediately: 'Coming! Give me two minutes!' Bruce's colleague was most amused. Sarah and I shared the Spanish language and would make it part of our daily life. We would translate into 'Spanglish' in a way that only people sharing the two languages would have appreciated."

Vanesa continues: "I'll never forget the skirts Sarah wore. They fascinated me, and we never saw that type of clothing in Buenos Aires. Only rarely did Sarah wear trousers and she always colour co-ordinated her clothes; they were never mis-matched.

"On another occasion Sarah came out to Argentina just with Mark, as this time they would be travelling round South America. I remember her sitting on the stairs muttering about her dream trip coming to nothing as Mark had had to return early to the UK. After Mark left, Richard and I went out practically every evening to chat and have a couple of drinks in different pubs round Belgrano, the district where the Brown family lives. Sarah was fascinated by the different wines, beers and champagnes. How we enjoyed chatting and killing ourselves laughing! Sarah and I – the same as our respective mothers – have a special noisy laugh... Brown style! *(Val, who translated this letter from Vanesa from Spanish into English, notes that she has left the 'have a special noisy laugh' in the present tense that Vanesa uses. This memory is so strong with her that it is as if Sarah is still around).*

"For a while during our college years we slightly lost touch, but we always talked to each other at Christmas, New Year, birthdays. Our mothers, the 'Brown sisters' did everything they could to ensure that we kept close, despite the distance between us. With the passage of time we became progressively closer. It is thanks to them that we had a more than special relationship and I feel more convinced than ever that nobody and nothing will be able to separate these two families who, despite adversity, keep seeing each other, talking and letter-writing. Over the years we kept writing and sending each other photos. We would tell each other secrets about our relationships, boyfriends and friends and acquaintances.

"In 1994 Oscar and I decided to marry in the following year. As this was a special occasion and as the family would be coming over from England for the event we decided that my aunt Val would be my husband's sponsor, and Sarah would be my registry office witness. (In Argentina the priest or minister cannot officiate legally; you always have to marry at the registry office, and if you so wish, follow with a wedding in a place of worship). According to Argentine law Sarah was not able to be my legal witness, though she took on this role in spirit. Because of this I decided she would give the principal reading from the Bible during the church service.

"It was very moving as Sarah read the words, without making a mistake, and in perfect Spanish. Having spent a considerable time living in Vigo she was able to speak fluent Spanish and it was lovely hearing her speak with that accent! I remember that at the wedding party she never stopped dancing. I always envied the way Sarah could dance.

"She had a perfect 'swing' just like Val. Everyone watched Sarah and commented how *simpatica* she was, and how well she danced. (*Simpatica* is a near-untranslatable word; it is better than charming, it means someone approachable, open-hearted, ready to talk).

"The first time I visited England with my daughter Maria Victoria I remember how Sarah played with and looked after my baby. On one occasion she asked if she could give Victoria her bath and I said of course she could. I told Sarah she didn't have to ask me first as Victoria was her niece. What Sarah categorically refused to do was change Victoria's nappies. No way would she do this. With the tact that was typical of Sarah she replied that this was one of the many tasks and obligations of a mother. I started laughing!"

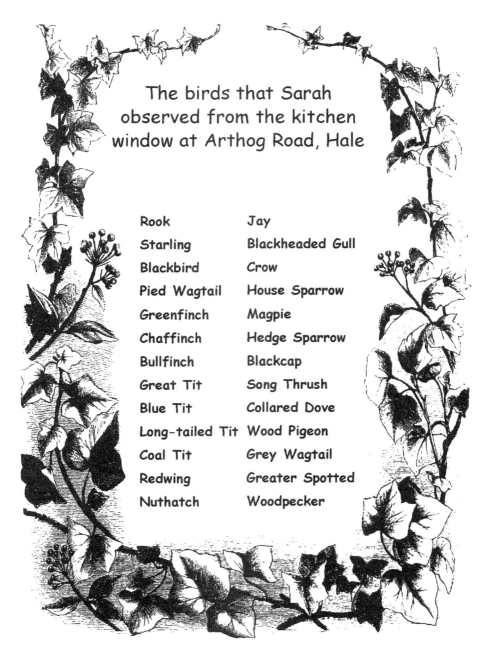

The birds that Sarah
observed from the kitchen
window at Arthog Road, Hale

Rook	Jay
Starling	Blackheaded Gull
Blackbird	Crow
Pied Wagtail	House Sparrow
Greenfinch	Magpie
Chaffinch	Hedge Sparrow
Bullfinch	Blackcap
Great Tit	Song Thrush
Blue Tit	Collared Dove
Long-tailed Tit	Wood Pigeon
Coal Tit	Grey Wagtail
Redwing	Greater Spotted
Nuthatch	Woodpecker

MUSIC THAT SARAH LOVED:
Nursery rhymes
Abba
Texas
Mercedes Sosa
Prince
The Chieftains
Oasis
Alison Moyet
Bach - B Minor Mass
The Verve
Mendelssohn - Elijah
Mansun
Ladysmith Black Mambazo
Handel - Messiah
Celiz Cruz
The Martyr Mantras
Youssou n'dour
Son Candela
Rossini - Petite Messe
John Lee Hooker
Juan Luis Guerra
Salsa
The Saw Doctors
Merengue
Fatboy Slim
Tom Jones
Macy Gray
Van Morrison
Christmas Carols
Talking Heads
The Pogues

THAT CHOCOLATE CAKE
Jane Ali-Knight, a school friend of Sarah:

"My first memories are not strictly of Sarah but of her Mum's wonderful chocolate cake which became legendary among the schoolgirls at Loreto...

"...then came our brief moment of fame together in 3Ji's acclaimed production of 'Toad of Toad Hall'. Sarah was well liked, and great fun, at school. She amazed me with her determination and will to succeed, even when we tried to lead her astray by inviting her to party the night away with us at discos in Warrington.

"After school Sarah and I lost touch again for a few years but when we met again at a Loreto reunion it was as if we'd seen each other yesterday. We chatted for hours. During the next few years our friendship grew and grew and Sarah became a very special and important friend to me. Whenever I think of her, I always recall happy positive times. Sarah shared my love of travel and adventure; I was fortunate enough to visit her in Spain and Portugal where I practised my Spanish, which was very basic compared with Sarah's! A love of the arts was another thing we shared. She was my cinema companion in Manchester and every year we attended the Edinburgh Festival together.

"Sarah was an amazing person, an incredible and loyal friend. She was always there for me, often as The Voice of Reason during difficult times. I was astounded by Sarah's positivity and love of life. In all the twenty two years I knew her I hardly ever saw her down, or unhappy. She was a wonderful presence at a dinner party as she loved being with people and could chat away effortlessly.

"During our friendship we spent time apart, fulfilling our wanderlust, but I still felt close to Sarah, especially as she was such a good correspondent. She was the one person who managed to attend all three of our wedding celebrations in the UK, and my biggest regret is that she didn't live to see the next generation of Ali-Knights.

"'Friends are for life'; Sarah was certainly in that category of friend. I feel very honoured to have known Sarah and to have had her as a close friend all those years. People like Sarah are very rare, and come along once in a person's lifetime. I have lost a very important person but the emptiness left by Sarah can be filled by my wonderful memories of her."

THE STRAIGHT A's
Liz Cochrane, a Loreto school friend:

"Towards the O level years Sarah emerged as one of those elite members of the year who always got straight A grades in her exams. Needless to say I was not in her class. In the language classes the clever ones did Latin, the mediocre did German, and the strugglers and the rebels did Spanish. I was only mediocre!

"I remember seeing Sarah in the library, looking at her A level notes condensed into a small box full of bubble charts etc. I had

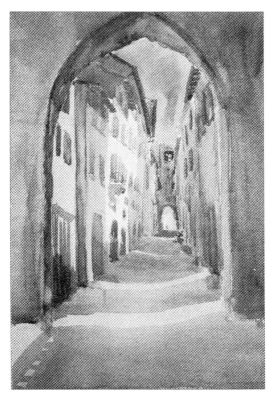

Painting by
Liz Cochrane

never seen anything like that. My notes were bursting out of two huge files and were intimidating just to look at!.

"Years later, when Sarah had returned from Spain and I had left my job in London we both ended up back in Manchester and our parents suggested we meet. I found that we were meeting at a crossroads of our lives. I was thinking about living in Italy. Sarah had just come back from Spain and was looking for the right job. We had more in common than we ever had at school.

"At this time I was going backwards and forwards to Italy but still feeling a bit aimless. Sarah was a good friend back in Manchester and we had some good talks about doing unconventional things with our lives and I will always be grateful for that. Sometimes when I have been unsure about my decision to live in Italy and getting out of the rat-race I remember Sarah and I remember to live my life to the full and enjoy it."

THE GIRL WITH THE AUBURN HAIR
John Walsh, former History Tutor, Jesus College, Oxford:
"As a university teacher I interviewed a great many would-be students, but my first impression of Sarah, from eighteen years ago, remains vivid; the lively girl from Altrincham, friendly and open, with a very nice sense of fun and a ready smile – and a sharp mind. With her impeccable A levels, A1, A, A, A, naturally we took her on board at Jesus College and she certainly deserved the Open Exhibition she was awarded.

"Going to university, crossing the bridge which is poised precariously between childhood and adulthood, can be anxiety-inducing for some, but Sarah did not seem to find it so. On the contrary, she simply enjoyed it. She had the good fortune to belong to a very friendly and tight-knit group of historians in her year. But even more, they had the great good fortune to have her as a friend. There was a lot of fun and laughter. Sarah, more than anyone, kept the group moving along happily together.

"On arrival Sarah was eager to try the good things on the university menu. She was not a scholarly recluse, not a fanatical athlete, not a good-time party girl, but the all-rounder who enjoyed work and play with equal zest. Her choices from the array of 'optional' courses on the Oxford history syllabus tell a story.

Many students focus cautiously on a particular period or even area, but Sarah was adventurous. In her intellectual time-capsule she liked to travel widely across the centuries. She picked topics as far apart as literature and society in sixteenth century England, late nineteenth century Europe, and a detailed 'special subject' on India under the Raj from 1919-1931. Quite a range!

"In tutorials she listened hard, but was generally combative too; one of those model students who take their teachers seriously – but not too seriously, and don't mind stropping their dialectical razors on their elders. In Finals she did well, with a good sprinkling of Alpha marks. Her essay on Women's' History in the General Paper seems particularly to have impressed the examiners, though I never dared ask what she wrote in it.

"Sarah took to student life, in all its aspects, like a duck to water. And take to the water she did. She took up college rowing, and loved it. She had a lot of energy. If she looked just a little like some auburn-haired ivory-skinned Pre-Raphaelite maiden from a Burne-Jones painting, she was very much tougher. Though far from beefy, she was strong and wiry enough to hold her own in the Women's' First Eight. From the balcony of the College boat house in 'Eights Week' one could see that red hair from far away, as her crew glided gracefully down the Thames in pursuit of a Bump.

"When I think of Sarah the adjectives that spring to mind are lively, funny, intelligent, kind.

"And perhaps another key word would be 'natural'. Her gaiety and intelligence seemed to bubble up inside her, clear, unforced, and unmediated, from the depths of her personality.

"Though students may not know it, when they 'go down' from Oxford, a very short report used to be concocted for them and kept in College, just in case it was needed suddenly for some job application when the tutors were away. Sarah's begins with the words, 'She was in all senses an asset to the college'. And that was what everyone here, friends, scouts or tutors, felt about Sarah Hotter. A golden girl whom we will always remember!"

DAWN CELEBRATION
Anne Fletcher recalls a Jesus College coach trip to the Granada

TV studios in Manchester in the spring of 1985. The college team won that year's final of *University Challenge*. Sarah and others had banners, and cheered the team on to success.

After the recording session, the coach returned through the night to Oxford, in time for Sarah and Anne to head straight down to Magdalen College to hear the singing of the college choir in the bell tower of the chapel. This performance is traditionally given at dawn, as a celebration of May Day. Anne well remembers the loveliness of this experience.

CANDLES, APLOMB AND ALCOHOL
Mary Simpson, formerly of ICL Personnel Department:

"I first met Sarah when I was in charge of the graduate recruitment programme for ICL. I was sent to conduct the 'milk-round' interviews at the Randolph Hotel in Oxford, and spent a day interviewing graduates.

"ICL's reputation was as a technical organisation, so the candidates were mostly computer science or physics graduates. However, we were trying to recruit people to work with customers as account support managers. They would work alongside sales people and other technical consultants, to understand the customer's requirements and then create a solution to meet those needs. We needed people with some technical understanding, but interpersonal skills were more important. Sarah rather stood out from the crowd!

"She was mature, and an excellent communicator and I had no hesitation in recommending her. However, it was not only these skills which left such a strong impression! She turned up for the interview looking extremely smart and professional, but carried a large bag with her, which she left by the door of the hotel room while we talked. After the formal interview, she mentioned that she was off to do some rowing or coxing – I cannot remember which. She asked if there was anywhere in the hotel where she could change, so, as I had time before the next candidate, she used the en-suite bathroom. She emerged looking slightly less smart than she had earlier, but she carried the whole thing off with her usual aplomb!

"I left personnel and moved across into sales, which is where I came across Sarah again, along with Andy, Chris, George and Miranda. We had a really tough task, breaking into a new marketplace, with woefully inadequate systems, but we all had a wonderful time working together! We would often share ideas. I organised a conference once to try and entice new customers to come and talk with us. The MP, Emma Nicholson, was doing a lot of work on Security of Information, and had worked for ICL before becoming an MP, so we approached her to speak at the event. I liaised with her secretary and Emma and I exchanged letters.

"However, about one week before the event, I was informed that Emma was totally deaf, something which no one had mentioned before! To the great amusement of the legal team, I was rather daunted by the prospect of a deaf speaker as I had no idea what practical issues this would raise. In fact Emma was a superb speaker and the only requirement she had was that I sat near the front to help with questions after her talk in case she couldn't see the speaker to lip-read. At the end of the evening I saw my colleagues, including Sarah, applauding me for my hard work but it took a long time for me to live that down!

"I also remember going to one of Sarah's parties when she was living in north London. There were loads of candles everywhere, and lots of alcohol! I went into London with Sarah once and saw a South American dance troupe.

"My overriding memories of Sarah are of someone with a tremendous sense of humour, and a person who was so kind and compassionate. We all took the mickey out of each other and the banter was fast and furious. Sarah was more than able to hold her own and join in, but it was never at the expense of anyone's feelings; she always knew that line between teasing someone and causing offence. She was a joy to work with."

MAKING THE CONNECTION
Rosemary McGee:
"In 1998 I was lodging with a friend of Sarah's and Sarah would often visit. She presented me one day with the latest Amnesty International magazine because featured in it were a Colombian

couple who'd been friends of mine but had been assassinated by paramilitaries in their flat in Bogota the previous year when I'd been living in Colombia. Sarah had learnt of this, had absorbed and retained it enough, and absorbed and retained every prisoner or assassination case enough to make the connection and give me the article. So many people, even if they'd noticed the article, might have shied away but Sarah knew I'd want to see it. In everything, she was a straight dealer.

"I remember the weekend she spent with me at my flat in London, November 1998 when she was already undergoing therapy for her brain tumour. She bowled me over with her positive energy and her stylish hat. We had a lovely lovely weekend of each other's company. Soon after she arrived I was putting lunch together. As we chatted madly, Sarah said 'Shall I toss the salad?' This she did, seamlessly continuing the flow of conversation, with a familiarity, a homeliness and a practicality and a respect for a good chat which shouldn't be interrupted. Now, I can't toss a salad without thinking of Sarah. It's lovely to have that reminder.

"I remember when I first met Sarah. I'd heard surprising and wonderful things about this woman who'd lived in Vigo, spoke good Spanish, and was even half-Argentinian. We met on a spring evening. We clicked at once, and talked and talked like old friends till long after I'd planned to go home. Infinitely practical, warm, immediate, quick-minded, with a touching and surprising eye for detail, and always ready to laugh. That's how I'd sum Sarah up."

I SHOULD HAVE WRIGGLED HARDER
David Parsons, a childhood friend of Valerie Hotter:

"I got to know Sarah ever so slightly when she and Mark were in Buenos Aires in 1997, staying with dear Maureen, Mono and family for a short while at 'Villa Despelote' ('Chaosville' – Val's sister Maureen's name for her household) but one couldn't help noticing what a beautiful *chica* (girl) she was, and how extremely intelligent.

"One evening, out of the blue, she was nice enough to invite me out, to go to the movies or dancing or something, I can't remember what. Unfortunately I had a previous engagement, out of which I could not wriggle at short notice, so I was unable to take up her very kind and original offer. I must confess that I was very touched and complimented by her kind thought and have always regretted not having 'wriggled harder '. From this you can pick up the fun part of Sarah which was such a huge part of her character – the idea of asking an older gentleman out dancing – lovely, I thought.

"Sarah was a truly beautiful person, in every regard. *Que Dios la tenga en su gloria!* (May God hold her in his glory!)"

AFFINITY
Loly Castro Chorro, a pupil of Sarah's at the English Language School in Vigo, Spain:

"I enrolled at the language school in October 1993. English was a completely new language for me. At first, Sarah struck me as very "English", but there was definitely something, her feelings – spirit – that told me there was a Latin/Argentine connection with us here in Spain, via her mother. It was obvious from the start that she wanted to become part of the Spanish way of life and she identified herself with Spanish society. The Argentine/Spanish roots were strongly present in her.

"Sarah became my special friend and visited us at home. She would help about the place and enjoyed my cooking. She was open and kind with everyone. We shared outings, read together, cried sometimes, danced, had fun – I never saw her cross. When her father died she lived with us for a while.

"The classes were wonderful; Sarah was very resourceful and would think of fun things to help us learn English. I don't want to remember her illness; I only want her fighting, adventurous and resourceful spirit to live on."

THE PROPER GLUE
Margaret Main, an Educational Craft Consultant who worked with Sarah at the Northwich Salt Museum:

"How did we meet? I rang Northwich Salt Museum and asked to speak to the Education Officer. 'Oh, you want Sarah!' Not 'Miss', but 'Sarah'. Nice.

"I wondered tentatively if she would like me to do any craft workshops at the Museum. We agreed to meet. She came to meet me for coffee before that first workshop I did. (I still have the invoice for it, 13 August 1996). For the workshop I told Sarah what I needed, insisting on BOSTIK glue, the proper fast-working one. Sarah duly got it!

"New to the Museum, I had researched its beginning as a Workhouse. I decided to make peg dollies, dressed in the costumes of the time. Sarah was enthusiastic. 'Don't worry', she said, 'I've got the glue.' But I did worry. I had been running craft workshops for over twenty years, and heard many promises 'I'll get it', or 'We have that', only to discover that the right glue was not available. Sarah made sure that it was.

"I need not have worried. Sarah got every smallest item that I'd requested. This was the first time ever that this had happened. It made such a difference. It made me feel valued. It showed me I could trust her. It was the start of being 'paid to do something I enjoyed'. It was the beginning of being charmed by Sarah too!

"Whenever she could Sarah popped in to help me. Fresh as a jonquil, neat, slender, and fun. She told me 'You do too much at home', and gave up her lunch hour to help me clean up.

"I felt Sarah's vitality and her optimism. At the beginning, not knowing her, I saw her as keen but frail. I worried that her job might prove too demanding for her. But she was hard-working, highly organised, and tough. And such a lovely person to work with. She worked with me and knew when to let me get on with things. She brought tea for me.

"One day as we were clearing away she was a bit brisker than usual. She said 'I must love you and leave you. My mother and my aunt are taking me to lunch'. 'Why didn't you say?', I demanded, 'Why didn't you leave me to do the clearing up?' 'It's all right; it's done now,' she said, and off she sped. Sarah also noted what time I arrived, and made sure I was paid for any extra time I put in. She fought my corner in a way I could not.

"The day I heard of her illness I was doing 'sticky painting'. I'd drawn huge dragons and we had PVA glue, paint, sequins, beads and glitter; all busy and bright, Fun to do, messy to clear away – without Sarah to help. I did not know that this workshop, which Sarah had set up, would bring her so strongly to mind. She was being hurried to hospital as we implemented her newest system

'Come any time, do it, take your work with you.' I felt odd being there without her, like a child coming home to an empty house.

"I sent her some pot-pourri I'd made, wondering whatever I could say to her mother, whom I have never met. I rang to see how Sarah was. Sarah answered the phone. She sounded her usual self, full of life, spring-like. I was both shaken and delighted. I invited her to my sixtieth birthday party and dance, and she came with her brother; smiling, funny, knowing no one but me, chubby-faced from the drugs. Cheerfully she informed me that she had to have another operation very soon. I was so pleased she'd come; I was never to see her again.

"Though I was able to talk once more to Sarah on the phone, it had to be a short chat. She was stumbling over words, and was clearly tired. It was the last time I spoke to her. When I put the phone down I felt very angry that someone so lovely and so valuable should have been stricken in this way. She had so much to give and her life had hardly begun. Surely there was a cure... but no. The Salt Museum telephoned me when she died and I was shocked that all her courage and our prayers had been in vain.

"Well Sarah, if you are watching, you will know that everyone who met you was drawn to you because you were simply lovely, right through. But I do wish I'd said so when you were here to tell."

THE SECOND SOPRANO

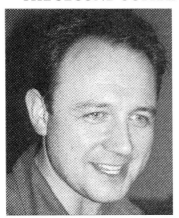

Steven Roberts *(pictured left)* is the Musical Director of the Altrincham Choral Society, which meets each week at Oak Road Methodist Church in Hale. The Choir gives public concerts at the Royal Northern College of Music in Manchester, with programmes planned up to two years ahead. During a rehearsal of Dvorak's *Stabat Mater,* I met Steven to talk about Sarah.

Val joined the Choir in 1995. She brought Sarah along in 1996, and

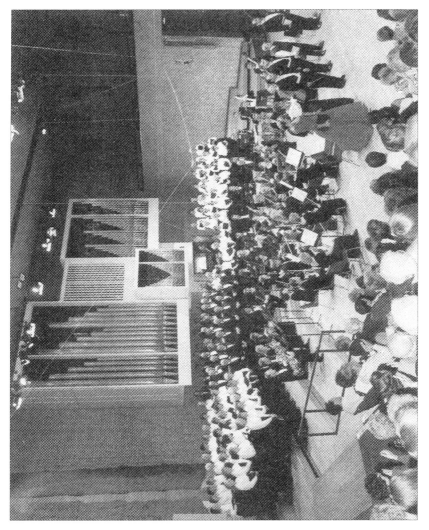

Altrincham
Choral Society:
Sarah was in the
Second
Sopranos.
(Photo by Karen
Wright for
Cheshire Life,
Oct 96, Vol 63,
No 10).

Sarah sang there right up to the date of her final admission to hospital in December 1999. It is customary for choirs to be subdivided into sections; Sarah was placed in the Second Sopranos. She had been in her school choir, and sang in the Oxford Bach Choir and her college choir when she was at university. She also joined choirs when she worked in London and later in Spain. Sarah was always singing round the house, and was well versed in popular music. She was au fait with the 'in' bands, Status Quo, Queen, etc., and who the instrumentalists were; Bruce, her father, had an extensive collection of records and CDs. Val, whose preference was more for classical music, often wished the sound of the 'pop' music could be turned down!

When Sarah came for the Altrincham Choir audition, she struck Steven Roberts as a very nice person. He remembers her lovely smile, her "alive communicative" face. This is a trait he likes in his members. Conductors give out a lot, and appreciate a response. Sarah's "aliveness" never faded, even when she was very ill. Notwithstanding a slight memory loss, Sarah sang in two Manchester concerts. She was a regular attender at rehearsals. There is a strong cameraderie in the Altrincham Choral Society; its members were well aware of the pressures Val and Sarah were under, and took them under its collective wing. For a period, Val and Sarah were absent from rehearsals. Steven did not know why, until they returned and told him simply that Sarah was "not well". When he asked what was the matter, they told him not to worry.

Steven speaks of Sarah's "charm, grace, interest and aura" – all transmitted naturally without her making any effort to impress. He was very touched when Val contacted him on Christmas Day 1999 to inform him of Sarah's death that morning and to request that he conduct the Choral Society at the funeral. Sarah had already chosen the items for the service, including three anthems by John Rutter, *The Lord is My Shepherd*, *For the Beauty of the Earth* and *The Lord Bless You and Keep You*.

Steven readily agreed to conduct the choral items at Sarah's funeral. All the Choir members were feeling very emotional. But Steven felt that, troubled though his feelings were, he had to provide a performance of the highest standard, especially for Sarah and her family. In this he succeeded.

Steven speaks about Sarah's spiritual gifts, her enjoyment of life, the diversity of her interests and concerns, "all the good work she was involved with." He admires Val for returning to rehearsals so soon after the funeral, especially as music is "sheer emotion".

How did Steven connect with Sarah's illness? He believes there is reason in adversity.

He had a young friend with cancer. The friend had a little daughter. Steven watched him. and wondered "Why him, and not me?" The friend gained tremendous strength from being ill. He changed from being insular to a person who really enjoyed life. Steven felt he could relate to what the friend was going through. And so it was with Val and Sarah. "To see someone with such strength in such a vulnerable position is a lesson for all of us."

THE DAILY LETTER
Melanie Preston:
Melanie met Sarah at Altrincham Choral Society. She recalls how Sarah's sense of humour stood her in good stead, and "made things easier for the rest of us when she was ill." After Sarah's final admittance to the Christie Hospital, Melanie sent a letter every day, which Val read to Sarah. Melanie says Sarah realised "this was it; but she wanted to make everyone else OK".

THE KNOCK AT THE DOOR
Maureen Mulholland, a family friend, was a great support to Sarah in her illness; a couple of times a week there would be a knock at the door and a smiling Maureen would come in, quite often accompanied by some cheering-up treat for Sarah. There was a black and white dog, a 'proper' Lakeland sheep, fluffy and comfortable, many toiletries and the woodpecker toy, which clacked its way down a steel support, making Sarah smile widely. Maureen says Sarah made it easy for friends, who might be feeling awkward or upset because of her illness, by her cheerful, down-to-earth approach. She recalls the Hotter Boxing Day parties, "where we were included in what was very much a family and old friends gathering, with games and feasting". These

A quotation from the poem entitled 'Warning' but commonly known as: 'When I Am Old I Shall Wear Purple':

"I shall sit down on the pavement when I'm tired
and gobble up samples in shops and press
alarm bells,
I shall go out in my slippers in the rain
And pick the flowers in other people's gardens,
And learn to spit."

Jenny Joseph

Sarah bought a tea towel with these lines from the poem on it while she and her mother were browsing at the Cheshire Fair and told the man at the stall that this was for her mother. The man said to Valerie, "You will have to learn how to spit." Valerie replied, "It's all right, my daughter has already taught me how to spit."

included Maureen's father, who came on several occasions. Although nonplussed by some of the games, he sometimes came into his own, coming up with a bizarre correct answer to a quiz question relating to his youth, as in a "Lanchester" car, which no one else had thought of.

HOT CHOCOLATE, AND A WALK WITH SHANTY
Ken Veitch:
"After Sarah had become ill, and had given up her work at the Salt Museum, I went to see her and Val at their home in Hale. I was treated to the usual Hotter hospitality. From our working days together, Sarah had remembered my liking for a mid-morning drink of hot chocolate. Carefully, but laboriously because of her condition, she set about making me one. Tasks that she would have done instinctively not long ago – opening the cupboard, selecting the mug, locating the chocolate, picking up the spoon – were now difficult and lengthy. All the time Val was on hand, ready to help if needed; the main thing was to keep Sarah achieving things, and give Sarah the positivity that followed from this. The hot chocolate was duly delivered to me; Sarah's solo effort. By now Sarah had a difficulty with numbers, and we signalled with fingers instead. But there was no embarrassment at all; everything was based on practicality and sense, and making Sarah's life as normal as possible. Our times together were relaxing and happy; I always left feeling better.

"With my daughters Lucy and Mary I help to look after a horse that lives about five miles from our home in Nantwich. His name is Shanty. He is a bay, with chestnut-coloured body and black mane and tail. We love grooming him, working with him in his paddock, and riding him along the quiet lanes; he is a very interesting and (usually!) well-behaved animal.

"During a visit to Val and Sarah I mentioned this as part of my news, and it was agreed that they would come to see Shanty for themselves. Our plan was to have lunch at home, then take Sarah for a short ride on Shanty.

"But I was shocked by Sarah's deterioration since I had last seen her. Her physical strength was much less. She struggled to find the simplest words. On that day – with the heroic unobtru-

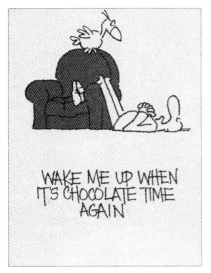
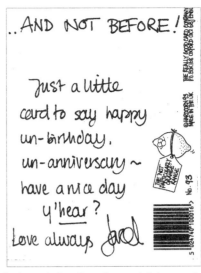

It wasn't only Ken Veitch who liked chocolate: Sarah sent this card to her mother. (Published by The Really Good Card Co., from 'The Not Particularly Orange' range)

sive support of Val, as ever – her illness was all too apparent. Yet we went ahead with our plan, as best we could. Sarah enjoyed gently brushing and stroking Shanty. Getting into the saddle, even with help, was beyond her, so instead Sarah led Shanty on a walk, from the stable down the drive to the lane and back, only about a hundred yards in all.

"Sarah's satisfaction was obvious, but the effort exhausted her. We drove back to the Veitch home in Nantwich, where she spent the afternoon asleep on Lucy's bed.

"That was the last time I saw Sarah. The lane where Shanty lives leads on to Beeston; from 'Woodpecker Corner' there is a lovely view across the fields towards the place where I met Sarah that first time in my office. I like to recall the merriment of that meeting, and to feel the essence of Sarah living on in the lives of us who knew her."

UPHELD

Patricia Lewis is a professional teacher of singing. For fifteen

132

years she was a mezzo-soprano with Opera North. She now lives in Northumberland. Patricia teaches in Manchester and Val is one of her pupils. Val asked if Sarah could have some lessons also. She told Patricia about Sarah's grave illness, and explained that the purpose of these lessons would be mainly therapeutic. Patricia agreed to take Sarah on. She remembers Sarah's bright personality, and, noting her singing voice, regrets she could not have worked with her earlier.

Their first meeting was at the Friends' (Quaker) Meeting House in Mount Street, Manchester, where Patricia hired a room. Patricia said a prayer each time Sarah was coming, and felt "upheld". She carefully chose songs that would be suitable for Val and Sarah separately. One lesson was immediately after a chemotherapy session that Sarah had undergone. It was Sarah who did the cheering up, urging her despondent mother to "Come on, woman, pull yourself together!"

One song that Patricia and Sarah enjoyed together was a bright, jazzy one, the last of a set of four traditional American songs – almost certainly of Negro origin – arranged by Michael Moores and entitled *Child of God*. The songs evoke the image of the Christ Child walking in the tree tops. They contain these lines.

If anyone asks you who I am
Tell them I'm a Child of God

If anyone asks you where I'm bound.
Tell them I'm bound for glory

EAGER BEAVER
Jane Hardman:
"When Sarah was taken ill she gladly entered into the spirit of such mad-cap ideas as "Why not become a golf pro?" Well why not! So the practice ground was soon witnessing a real eager beaver, thrashing away at the immobile, tantalising, white inch and a half THING on the tee peg. After a while the swing really began to develop and she got her eye in, as they say, and was hitting the ball a good 100 yards and more.

"We had some laughs – golf is nothing if not totally ridiculous, but it is such fun and it is good for you to be outside taking gentle exercise. This Sarah and I did, with a few excursions to the 19th too!"

A LETTER FROM NEUROSUREON JAMES LEGGATE
to Val Hotter, 11 February 2000:
"Dear Mrs Hotter

"I have only just been notified that Sarah was admitted to the Christie Hospital just before Christmas and sadly died on Christmas Day. Please accept that my thoughts and prayers are very much with you and your son. Sarah had put up a tremendous fight and had impressed me with her immense bravery as well as her sense of humour and thoughtfulness towards others during the time that I was privileged to look after Sarah.

"Her death will have left a huge hole in your lives, especially coming on so soon after the loss of your husband and there will be times when you wonder whether you can go on. It is at those sort of times that you need to remind yourself just what a powerful influence for good Sarah's life has been to all the people that she has touched. We none of us know the reason why we are put here on this earth in our own particular circumstances but I know that you, like Sarah, share a faith that will support you through the dark times as well as sustaining you through the good times.

"I am sure there will be times when you will feel rage and anger and frustration at the injustice of what you have suffered and of what Sarah has suffered, and these are all entirely normal emotions. There will also be times when you will question how these things started, how things might have turned out if Sarah had had different treatment at different times, and if I can help at any time just by being a listening ear or trying to answer some of your questions please do not hesitate to contact me. Sometimes, however, coming back to the hospital where your loved ones have been treated proves too painful an experience and I will quite understand and please be assured that this letter needs no reply."

Val Hotter notes:

James Leggate is a wonderful doctor, totally dedicated to his work.

One morning dressed in his operating clothes, he spent forty five min-
utes talking to Sarah and me. I am writing this to show my admiration
for the doctors. In trying to help Sarah they left no stone unturned.
James's comment, when I asked about any other possible treatment for
her was "Mrs Hotter, you have my word (he emphasised "word") that if
there is anything out there that would help Sarah, I'd make sure she
would have it."

VAL'S REPLY TO JAMES LEGGATE'S LETTER
19 March 2000:
"Dear James,

"I have a theory, not seriously thought out, just instinct, which I used when Bruce my husband died, that the right moment comes to do something, and don't worry about it till this time comes. This is such a moment, the time to reread again your lovely letter written last month about Sarah, and to thank you so much for your words. Your letter moved me deeply and it is yet another tribute to this wonderful daughter of mine, that so long after we saw you, you have been so affected by her life and now her death. At the time I did wonder whether you knew and felt that you would get to know via inter-hospital information.

"I will never forget our last meeting, when she was still well but we felt the warning signs during our conversation. You were always very kind with her and myself even though one knew that we were dealing with something so serious. Although one always hopes, over the last few months these warnings became very much part of our daily life. First her peripheral vision started to be affected, then her speech slowly lessened and later her walking became difficult. This is one of those occasions 'the spirit is willing but the flesh is weak'. Well, Sarah had no weakness about her insofar as the spirit was concerned. The flesh got beaten by her terrible illness but to the end her spirit was totally undimmed. Hers was a remarkable achievement; she never lost her smile and she developed a God-given patience and resourcefulness as well as her habitual cheerfulness. She never seemed outwardly to be out of control of the situation, even to the end, and although communication became so difficult she still very much knew her mind, and what she wanted. The courageous and cheerful way in which she handled her illness has had a major impact on people with whom she came into contact. This 'inspiration' is the continual message I have read in the many letters my son Mark and I have received. St Vincent's church in Altrincham was packed to overflowing on 7th January when we made our good-byes to Sarah. Everyone was very impressed with the number of people who came to share the occasion.

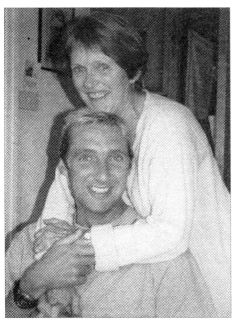

Val and Mark

"Sarah was taken into Christie Hospital the evening of 8th December and Mark and I were able to be with her all the time till she slipped away early Christmas morning. The ward staff accommodated us in Sarah's room and made sure we had everything we needed. We surrounded Sarah with the things that were important to her, and made her room as much a home as we could. We played music constantly; there was a radio, a CD player and a tape player. We took one of the pictures from Sarah's room here at home, and some of her ornaments and soft toys. There were many visitors, masses of flowers, cards, letters, baskets of fruit. We managed things in as ordinary way as we could. There was no drama, just lots of love and cuddles. The attention, respect and affection shown by the Christie staff was second to none. They were lovely with her and treated her so gently and with such consideration. Mark and I will always be grateful for this.

"Strangely you said something very important in your letter. It may be that you saw something in Sarah, I don't know, despite the few times we met, but you used the words 'powerful influence for good'. I have thought of those words many a time, because as I have said, things Sarah has said and done, and conversations with friends, have had a deep impact on many people, very often changing their lives, or the direction of their future lives. It doesn't make it any easier to live without her, but Mark and I feel a big sense of pride and strength from what she has done. I thought you might like a copy of what Sarah's friend Caron said in her tribute at the funeral.

"I feel, on reflection, that some people can pack a huge life into their lives. This life may be short, but Sarah's impact on many many people has been quite profound. This includes Mark, who of course has been deeply affected and who is also thinking of making changes to his own life.

"Sarah once said 'you have to allow people to do what they feel is right'; this is a good lesson. Whether one may or may not think something is right, or appropriate; if the other person feels it is right, that is good enough. One of her friends said to me that he felt that Sarah would want her friends to look after me. Whether or not I feel that this would be appropriate is not important. I remember what Sarah said and I accept their affection, allowing them to do what they feel is correct. Many of her friends still keep in touch with me. They are deeply shocked, I know; it is never easy for a young person to lose a friend of their own age. Sarah was always so bright and cheerful and such an enthusiast for life, that her friends are missing her company.

"I don't think I will want to come back to the hospital. I don't believe that there are unanswered questions. I just hope and pray that this awful illness will one day be beaten.

"In the meantime, good people like yourself and Dr Rao, who were so kind to Sarah, make it easier to bear."

A FIGHTER
A recollection by Sarah's cousin Richard:
"I find it difficult to write about Sarah. Despite time and distance we connected in a special way. Whenever we got together we never wanted to break it off. Sarah loved going out, sitting in some bar or other, or sitting under a tree in some park to chat for

hours. I remember us going out and about Buenos Aires on my motorbike, which Sarah loved. She loved observing people, how they interacted, how they were dressed. She loved nature, the flowers in the parks, watching the birds. She enjoyed being with people and was very *simpatica*, always smiling and talking the hind-leg off a donkey.

"She was always in good spirits and being with her was great fun. I remember Sarah as someone who had an insatiable curiosity, in the best sense of the word, always wanting to learn about things. She was a very extroverted person but never dwelt on herself. It was lovely being with her. But what affected me most deeply was seeing her as a real fighter, someone who would never back off from a problem. I think we all realised this at the end."

THE WEDDING OF JACKIE AND MIKE
A special journey:

On 4 December 1999, Sarah's friends Jackie and Mike married at Glendevon, a small village in central Scotland. Sarah and Val were invited. The weather was severe, with rain, snow and gales. A large tree had been blown down across the Hotters' garden in Hale, and there were floods. Though Sarah by this time had less than a month to live, she remained in good spirits, and very keen to be present at the wedding, With a three hundred mile car journey in prospect, Val checked the weather forecast. It was dire; the advice was not to travel unless absolutely necessary. However, the decision was taken to set off.

On the M6 the carriageway was down to one lane in places. Overturned lorries were seen at regular intervals. Looking back, Val feels that a cup of tea and biscuits, sitting comfortably and warmly at home, would have been much easier! But they were absolutely determined to press on, and eight hours later arrived at the Roman Camp Hotel at Callander, the village about fifteen miles north-west of Stirling, made famous by the *Dr Finlay's Casebook* TV series.

After their difficult journey, Val and Sarah were delighted to find such a luxurious and comfortable hotel. The place was decorated for Christmas, with plaids, tartans, ribbons, white heather and holly. There was the aroma of haggis cooking in the

Extracts from a poem for Sarah
by Peter Brennan:

SARAH

Trees were bare
Leaves all gone
Stark against the afternoon sun
The sky grey and intimidating
The wind making it all of a struggle

And yet we met in Spring last year
When darkness had come down
In that time in Ireland
But hope and help were sound

I fight and fight again
That is the Hotters' claim
But here I fight an enemy
Of whom I feel but cannot see

The Summer comes with flowers and trees
The Sunshine giving reason to please
And in the garden with Mummy
I share the work and love

kitchen. That evening there was a meal, lovely to eat and beautifully presented, with little bowls of tasty starters, five or six courses, and lots of fun and laughter.

The next morning the magic continued. Val and Sarah looked out of their window to see everywhere blanketed with snow. But the Scots are efficient at keeping their key roads open, and Val and Sarah had little trouble reaching the small stone church at Glendevon for the wedding service of Jackie and Mike. The hymns were *Praise My Soul, the King of Heaven*, and *Love Divine, All Loves Excelling*. Val describes the service as "very personal".

Returning to the hotel at Callander, Val and Sarah spotted a turning that the others missed. The others got tangled in the snow. Eventually everyone was together for a lovely reception, including another excellent meal. Sarah revelled in the food and the company.

She was with people she loved, and this was the way she wanted to spend the time that was left to her. She would go to great lengths – as she and Val had shown – to be with people she was fond of.

The ride home was much easier, with sunshine and clear blue skies. In five hours Val and Sarah were back in Hale. It was to be the last excursion that Sarah would make.

JUNE'S RAFFLE TICKETS
Coincidence?
Val writes: "Here is a message from my good friend June Colvill Jones. June lives in Argentina. We were at school together and the story of how she came to be with us when Sarah was taken into hospital is quite incredible.

"June had been saying for months before, 'You don't know how frustrated people are feeling here, that they are so far away and can't be near you to help.' Then one fine day she and her sister went to a garden fair and June bought some raffle tickets, as one does. The next morning she was rung up to be told she had won first prize, and the prize was a return flight to Amsterdam on KLM. When she rang KLM to organise a connecting flight to Manchester the lady on the other end of the phone was a distant relative of mine, who not only organised the connecting flight but when June arrived at Buenos Aires airport she was upgraded to Business Class and travelled in style!

"Having June here when we had that awful emergency was so wonderful; June was so helpful and supportive. I think it helped her, too, to feel that she had helped and maybe had represented all those loving people out there who couldn't be here at that time."

JUNE'S MESSAGE TO VAL

"My contact with Sarah was limited to her few trips to Argentina, and then the last days with her in December 1999. What I would like to say is that maybe you could use some of her fantastic written memories of her trip in Latin America with Mark, how she waited for Mark while he went back to the UK for the funeral of his girl-friend's mother and the loving friendship and companionship that was always evident between her and Mark.

"While I stayed with you in December 1999 I was struck by the constant stream of telephone messages for Sarah, the letterbox overflowing with cards and letters, and then when she was in hospital and I was at your home, the way the telephone rang, and how the answer-phone message box got filled up immediately with more calls whenever the house was empty for a short while.

"In other words, if God is Love, and love is shown through our 'neighbours', i.e. 'Thou shalt love thy neighbour as thyself', then the love that came pouring out for Sarah from all around the world was a manifestation of God's love for us."

WARD 3, THE CHRISTIE HOSPITAL, DECEMBER 1999
Sarah's final days, recalled by Sister Tina Johnson:

"Sarah was admitted to our ward on the evening of 8th December and was given the side room as her family wished to stay with her.

"From the outset they made that little room their home, a haven from the world. Our recollections of Sarah, Val and Mark are of a family as one with itself and at peace with the world.

"The room, in the initial days, often rang with laughter from the interaction of the frequent visitors, who were many and varied. As Sarah became less well, the visitors still came, but for shorter lengths of time, to sit with Sarah and chat quietly with her Mum and brother.

"Some of the memories, which remain with us, are:
• The radio/cassette playing favourite programmes and music
• The postcards and cards on display in the room
• A picture in place of the ward clock
• Photos of Sarah's travels and family
• Sarah's lovely auburn air and pale complexion
• The teddy bears sitting on the coloured handmade blanket on the bed
• The phone calls from friends unable to visit
• The flowers and attractive gifts for Sarah
• The subdued lighting and pleasant aromas

"We particularly remember Sarah's determination to continue as normal for as long as possible. With the help of her family she was able to achieve this until shortly before her death.

"Val and Mark assisted with all Sarah's physical care with only minimal support from the nursing staff.

"Val's husband had died quite recently and this must have made the family's acceptance of Sarah's death more difficult. None of us can recall a bitter comment from Sarah, Val or Mark as to why Sarah should suffer in this way and the family unit again be shattered.

"One nurse remembers talking with Val just before Christmas and learning that both she and Sarah were members of the Altrincham Choral Society. The previous year the nurse had been to their concert in Tatton Hall and bought their tape of Christmas music. She was delighted to discover that Sarah was singing on the tape. She told Val that she would treasure that tape and would play it every Christmas and think of them – and she does.

"Sarah's life finally drew to a close early on Christmas morning with Val and Mark supporting her to the end. The day a loved one dies always leaves a difficult memory for future anniversaries. If it happens on an already 'special day' such as Christmas, it must make it harder to cope with in the future.

"Val and Mark remained calm and 'strong' in their grief and were supportive to nursing staff who were also distressed at Sarah's death.

"One nurse recalls Val saying that she considered it a privilege that Sarah, the same age as Jesus when he died, had died on his birthday.

"The nurses caring for Sarah after her death felt desperately sad for Val and Mark at the loss of their loved one and sorry that Sarah had not been given the opportunity to fulfil her potential and achieve her desires for life.

"The nursing staff found it difficult working Christmas Day. Several of our patients were aware of Sarah's death. Also we knew, and many of them knew, that this was probably their last Christmas Day too. This made it difficult for us to summon up the *joie de vivre* that Sarah would have wished us to have that day.

"For one of the nurses caring for Sarah after her death on Christmas Day, it was also her birthday. Each year that day holds a tinge of sadness as she remembers the vital exuberance of Sarah.

"During those final dark days of Sarah's illness, Val and Mark seemed to be sustained and comforted by their strong faith in God. Although they may have questioned Sarah's illness inwardly they came over as accepting this challenge in life.

"Until almost her life's end Sarah manifested her love of life and her sense of fun. She was a shining light for a short time in our lives and some of her glow has surely remained with us for ever."

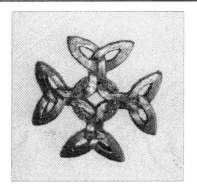

BLESSING
ON SETTING FORTH

MAY THE ROAD RISE TO MEET YOU.

MAY THE WIND ALWAYS BE AT
YOUR BACK.

MAY THE SUN SHINE WARM UPON
YOUR FACE,

THE RAINS FALL SOFT UPON YOUR
FIELDS;

AND, UNTIL WE MEET AGAIN, MAY
GOD HOLD YOU IN THE PALM
OF HIS HAND.

Traditional Celtic blessing

A CHARACTERISTIC COMMAND...

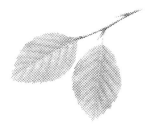

Dear Mummy ~

Happy Mother's Day

Forget the ironing. Ignore the
mess the kitchen is in (?) Don't
look at the carpets or investigate
the laundry bag. Forget the sorr-
ows. Ban any one else from 'booking'
the TV and plonk for the day.
By Order.

From Sarah at Oxford to Val, Mother's Day, 1986

ACKNOWLEDGEMENTS

Sarah Bate, Regional Appeals Officer, Christie Hospital, Manchester
Christopher Brandt, Colleague of Sarah, ICL Computers, London
Peter Brennan, Friend of Sarah at Altrincham
Vanesa Cabaña, Buenos Aires, Argentina, cousin of Sarah
Loly Castro Chorro, Language student in Vigo, Spain
Liz Cochrane, School friend of Sarah, Loreto Convent Grammar School
June Colville-Jones, Buenos Aires, school friend of Val in Argentina
Beth 'Auntie Beff' Crump, Friend of the Hotter family in Ashford, Kent
Frances Edwards, Artist, Northwich
Tessa Flood, Friend of the Hotter family in Ashford, Kent
Miiranda Freeman, Colleague of Sarah, ICL Computers, London
H Rao Gattamaneni, Consultant Clinical Oncologist, Christie Hospital
Sister Patricia Goodstadt, Head Teacher, Loreto Convent Grammar School
Jane Hardman, Friend of the Hotter family in Altrincham
Ann Hotter, Vancouver, Canada, Sarah's aunt
Kay Hobday, Press Officer, Bristol Cancer Help Centre
Jesus College, Oxford, Kind permission to use illustration
Tina Johnson, Sister, Ward 3, Christie Hospital
Martine Knoderer, Strasbourg, France, Sarah's pen-pal
James Leggate, Consultant Neurosurgeon, Hope Hospital, Salford
Patricia Lewis, Sarah's singing teacher
Andy Long, Colleague of Sarah, ICL Computers, London
Andrea Lyons, Teacher of languages and Sarah's flat mate in Vigo, Spain
Valda MacDonald, Colleague of Sarah, Salt Museum Education Dept
Margaret Main, Educational Craft Consultant, Northwich
Frances McGee, Deputy Head Teacher, and Sarah's history teacher, Loreto
John and Maureen Mulholland, Friends of the Hotter family in Hale
Anne O'Brien, Colleague of Sarah, Salt Museum Education Dept
David Parsons, Friend of the Hotter family in Buenos Aires, Argentina
Melanie Preston, Altrincham Choral Society
Steven Roberts, Musical Director, Altrincham Choral Society
Shirley Starkey, Colleague of Sarah, Salt Museum Education Dept
Anne (Fletcher) Teckman, Student friend of Sarah at Jesus College, Oxford
Frances Turner, Friend of the Hotter family in Ashford, Kent
Bernadette Turtle, Loreto Community, Llandudno
Maxine (Pillinger) Vaughan, Colleague of Sarah at ICL Computers, London

ACKNOWLEDGEMENTS

Caron (Leech) Walker, Friend of Sarah at Loreto Convent Grammar School
John Walsh, Sarah's History Tutor at Jesus College, Oxford
Carol Watts, Colleague of Sarah at Salt Museum Education Dept
Sheila Whitelegg, Friend of the Hotter family in Altrincham

We are also grateful to those who have allowed us to use copyright material in this book. Where we have been unable to establish contact with the copyright holder to obtain their permission, we have done our best to attribute the work to them.